CONTENTS

KT-553-851

LIST OF ABBREVIATIONS

ACh	Acetylcholine
AChE	Acetylcholinesterase
ACTH	Adrenocorticotrophic hormone
ADH	Antidiuretic hormone
ADP	Adenosine diphosphate
ALT	Alanine aminotransferase
ANP	Atrial natriuretic peptide
ANS	Autonomic nervous system
APTT	Activated partial thromboplastin time
ARDS	Adult respiratory distress syndrome
AST	Aspartate aminotransferase
ATP	Adenosine triphosphate
AV	Atrioventricular
AVP	Arginine vasopressin
BBB	Blood-brain barrier
BMR	Basal metabolic rate
BP	Blood pressure
cAMP	Cyclic adenosine monophosphate
CAT	Choline acetyl transferase
CBF	Coronary blood flow
CCK	Cholecystokinin
cGMP	Cyclic guanosine monophosphate
CNS	Central nervous system
CO	Cardiac output
COPD	Chronic obstructive pulmonary disease
CPAP	Continuous positive airway pressure
CRTZ	Chemoreceptor trigger zone
CSF	Cerebrospinal fluid
CVP	Central venous pressure
DAG	Diacylglycerol
DCT	Distal convoluted tubule
DHEA	Dehydroepiandrosterone
DOPA	Dihydroxyphenylalanine
ECF	Extracellular fluid

ECG/EKG	Electrocardiogram
EGF	Epidermal growth factor
EPSP	Excitatory postsynaptic potential
ERV	Expiratory reserve volume
FiO_2	Fraction of inspired oxygen
FEV	Forced expiratory volume
FFA	Free fatty acid
FRC	Functional residual capacity
FVC	Force vital capacity
GDP	Guanosine diphosphate
GFR	Glomerular filtration rate
GTP	Guanosine triphosphate
HCT	Haematocrit
IC	Inspiratory capacity
ICF	Intracellular fluid
IP_2	Inositol diphosphate
IP_3	Inositol triphosphate
IPSP	Inhibitory postsynaptic potential
IRV	Inspiratory reserve volume
IVC	Inferior vena cava
MAP	Mean arterial pressure
MEN	Multiple endocrine neoplasia
MI	Myocardial infarction
NMJ	Neuromuscular junction
NO	Nitric oxide
PAH	Para-aminohippuric acid
PAP	Pulmonary artery pressure
PCT	Proximal convoluted tubule
PDGF	Platelet-derived growth factor
PNS	Parasympathetic nervous system
PT	Prothrombin time
PVR	Pulmonary vascular resistance
R-A-A	Renin-angiotensin-aldosterone
RBF	Renal blood flow
RES	Reticuloendothelial system
RPF	Renal plasma flow

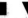

RV	Residual volume
SA	Sinoatrial
SIADH	Syndrome of inappropriate ADH
SLE	Systemic lupus erythematosus
SNS	Sympathetic nervous system
SR	Sarcoplasmic reticulum
SVR	Systemic vascular resistance
TCA	Tricarboxylic acid
TLC	Total lung capacity
TLV	Total lung volume
TSH	Thyroid-stimulating hormone
TV	Tidal volume
VC	Vital capacity
V/Q	Ventilation/perfusion ratio

LIST OF ABBREVIATIONS

To my daughter, Edel Roya Kanani

PREFACE

A well-known doctor once told me that "learning is the noblest form of begging". This is certainly what it feels like just before the MRCS exam when the brain labours with the weight of temporary information. Physiology is not an inherently difficult subject – only made so by the unholy trinity of a bad night on-call, dwindling time and a thick textbook. I hope that this book is the remedy to this unfortunate combination, and helps a little to play the game.

M.K
M.J.E
January 2004

A CHANGE IN POSTURE

Below is a set of graphs showing some cardiovascular parameters during a change in posture from supine to standing, and then to supine again.

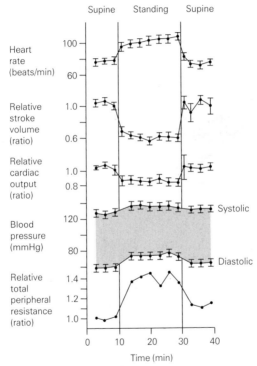

From Smith J, Bush J, Weidmeier V and Tristani. Application of impedance cardiography to study of postural stress. Journal of Applied Physiology, 29:133. The American Physiological Society, 1970

1. What happens to the stroke volume when standing up after a period of lying supine? Explain why this change occurs

Standing up increases the venous pooling of blood in the most dependent parts of the body. (Veins are, after all, capacitance vessels.) This redistribution of blood causes a reduction in the intrathoracic blood volume returning to the heart. Through the Frank-Starling mechanism, this causes a reduction in the stroke volume (by 30–40%). This rises again when going back to the supine position, in response to increased venous return.

2. What happens to the arterial pressure during this period?

Despite changes in the physiologic environment and stroke volume, reflex responses ensure that there is little change in the arterial pressure.

3. What is the physiologic relationship between the cardiac output (CO) and the arterial pressure normally?

The arterial pressure is defined as the product of the CO and the systemic vascular resistance (SVR) and may be considered as the *afterload*. An increase of this places a negative feedback on any further rise in the CO.

4. What physiologic mechanisms ensure that the arterial pressure is maintained after standing?

The changes that occur may be understood by considering the relationship of the arterial pressure to the heart rate and SVR.

Arterial pressure = CO × SVR

where CO = heart rate × stroke volume

∴ Arterial pressure = heart rate × stroke volume × SVR

There is a fall in the stroke volume, so in order to maintain the blood pressure (BP), the heart rate and the SVR must *increase*

- Carotid baroreceptor stimulation is reduced following a fall in the pulse pressure on standing.

▼

This causes a reduction of vagal cardiac stimulation, and an increase in sympathetic nervous system (SNS) stimulation of the heart and peripheral vasculature

- There is, therefore, an increase in the heart rate by 15–20 beats per minute
- Increased peripheral SNS activity stimulates arteriolar vasoconstriction – increasing the SVR
- There is also some venoconstriction, limiting the amount of peripheral blood pooling
- There is a sympathetically-mediated inotropic effect on the myocardium, limiting the fall in the stroke volume and CO
- As a result of increases in the heart rate and SVR, the arterial pressure may actually rise slightly on standing

5. Give some common causes for postural hypotension.

- *Failure to increase the CO during standing*
  - Simple vaso-vagal syncope
  - Fixed heart rate or bradycardia: β-blockers, heart block, sick sinus syndrome
  - Myocardial diseases: cardiomyopathy, other cardiac failure
- *Reduced stroke volume*
  - Fixed afterload: aortic stenosis, pulmonary embolism
  - Dehydration, diuretics
- *Reduced SVR*
  - Vasodilator drugs, e.g. α-blockers, nitrates, antidepressants
  - Pregnancy
  - Sepsis
  - Autonomic failure, e.g. chronic diabetes mellitus

ACID-BASE

1. Define the pH.
The pH is $-\log_{10}[H^+]$.

2. What is the pH of the blood?
7.36–7.44.

3. Where does the H^+ in the body come from?
Most of the H^+ in the body comes from CO_2 generated by metabolism. This enters solution, forming carbonic acid through a reaction mediated by the enzyme carbonic anhydrase.

$$CO_2 + H_2O \rightleftharpoons H_2CO_3 \rightleftharpoons H^+ + HCO_3^-$$

Acid is also generated by
- Metabolism of the sulphur-containing amino acids cysteine and methionine
- Anaerobic metabolism, generating lactic acid
- Generation of the ketone bodies: acetone, acetoacetate and β-hydroxybutyrate

4. What are the main buffer systems in the intravascular, interstitial and intracellular compartments?
In the *plasma* the main systems are:

- The bicarbonate system
- The phosphate system ($HPO_4^{2-} + H^+ \rightleftharpoons H_2PO_4^-$)
- Plasma proteins
- Globin component of haemoglobin

Interstitial: the bicarbonate system
Intracellular: cytoplasmic proteins.

5. What does the Henderson–Hasselbalch equation describe, and how is it derived?
This equation, which may be applied to any buffer system, defines the relationship between dissociated and

undissociated acids and bases. It is used mainly to describe the equilibrium of the bicarbonate system.

$$CO_2 + H_2O \rightleftharpoons H_2CO_3 \rightleftharpoons H^+ + HCO_3^-$$

The dissociation constant,

$$K = \frac{[H^+][HCO_3^-]}{[H_2CO_3]}$$

Therefore

$$[H^+] = K \frac{[H_2CO_3]}{[HCO_3^-]}$$

Taking the $\log_{10}$

$$\log_{10}[H^+] = \log_{10} K + \log_{10} \frac{[H_2CO_3]}{[HCO_3^-]}$$

Taking the negative log, which expresses the pH, and where $-\log_{10}K$ is the pK

$$pH = pK - \log_{10} \frac{[H_2CO_3]}{[HCO_3^-]}$$

Invert the term to remove the minus sign:

$$pH = pK + \log_{10} \frac{[HCO_3^-]}{[H_2CO_3]}$$

The $[H_2CO_3]$ may be expressed as $pCO_2 \times 0.23$, where 0.23 is the solubility coefficient of CO_2 (when the pCO_2 is in kPa).

The pK is equal to 6.1.

▼

Thus,

$$pH = 6.1 + \log_{10} \frac{[HCO_3^-]}{pCO_2 \times 0.23}.$$

6. Which organ systems are involved in regulating acid-base balance?

The main organ systems are:

- *Respiratory system:* this controls the pCO_2 through alterations in the alveolar ventilation. Carbon dioxide indirectly stimulates central chemoceptors (found in the ventro-lateral surface of the medulla oblongata) through H^+ released when it crosses the blood-brain barrier (BBB) and dissolves in the cerebrospinal fluid (CSF)
- *Kidney:* this controls the $[HCO_3^-]$, and is important for long-term control and compensation of acid-base disturbances
- *Blood:* through buffering by plasma proteins and haemoglobin
- *Bone:* H^+ may exchange with cations from bone mineral. There is also carbonate in bone that can be used to support plasma HCO_3^- levels
- *Liver:* this may generate HCO_3^- and NH_4^+ (ammonia) by glutamine metabolism. In the kidney tubules, ammonia excretion generates more bicarbonate

7. How does the kidney absorb bicarbonate?

There are three main methods by which the kidneys increase the plasma bicarbonate:

- Replacement of filtered bicarbonate with bicarbonate that is generated in the tubular cells
- Replacement of filtered phosphate with bicarbonate that is generated in the tubular cells
- By generation of 'new' bicarbonate from glutamine molecules that are absorbed by the tubular cell

8. Define the base deficit.

The base deficit is the amount of acid or alkali required to restore 1 l of blood to a normal pH at a pCO_2 of 5.3 kPa and at 37°C. It is an indicator of the metabolic component to an acid-base disturbance. The normal range is -2 to $+2$ mmol/l.

ACTION POTENTIALS

1. What is meant by the 'equilibrium potential' for an ion?

The equilibrium potential of an ion is the potential difference at which that ion ceases to flow down its electrochemical gradient across the cell membrane. It is calculated by the *Nernst* equation.

2. What is meant by the 'resting membrane potential' for a cell?

This is the potential difference across the cell membrane. This occurs due to the ionic fluxes of Na^+, K^+, and Cl^- across the membrane, the sizes of which are determined by their electrochemical gradients. It is calculated by the *Goldman* equation, which takes into account the contribution of the equilibrium potentials of each species of ion that crosses the membrane.

3. What is the typical value of the resting membrane potential for a neurone?

A typical value is $-70\,mV$. The value is negative because the interior of the cell is negatively charged with respect to the exterior.

4. What is the importance of the Na^+/K^+ pump for the equilibrium potential?

This pump, which is ATPase-driven, transports 3 Na^+ out of the cell for 2 K^+ pumped in. It helps to maintain the internal and external ionic environment that progressively alters as ions naturally flow down their electrochemical gradients. In doing so, it maintains and sustains the potential difference across the cell (Resting membrane potential).

5. What is an action potential? Draw and label the axes of a typical action potential for a neurone.

This is defined as the rapid change in the membrane potential (depolarisation) that occurs following stimulation of an excitable cell. It is followed by a rapid return to the resting membrane potential (repolarisation).

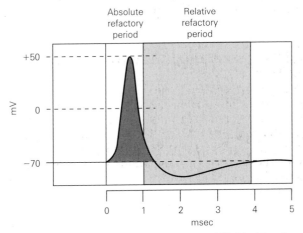

Reproduced with permission from Berne RM, Levy MN. Principles of Physiology, 3rd edition, 2000, London, with permission from Elsevier

- Note that depolarisation is an 'all-or-none' response, in that the action potential is generated only when the threshold potential is reached by the stimulus. Sub-threshold stimuli do not generate the action potential
- For any individual excitable cell, each action potential is of the same amplitude, and propagated at the same speed

6. Briefly describe the ionic basis for the action potential.

The changes in the fluxes of ions that account for depolarisation may be summarised in the following graph:

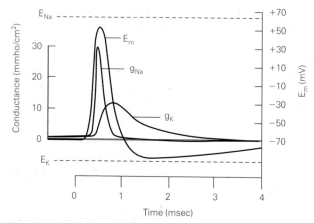

Where E_m = Membrane potential
From Berne RM, Levy MN. Principles of Physiology, 3rd edition, 2000, London, with permission from Elsevier

- Once the threshold potential is reached by the stimulus, the voltage-sensitive Na^+-channels open, causing a rapid influx of Na^+ into the cell. This causes depolarisation, and the membrane potential becomes positive. Once open, the Na^+-channel closes again within milliseconds
- During the initial opening of the Na^+-channels, a positive feedback loop is initiated; so more channels open up, leading to rapid depolarisation
- The cell would remain depolarised if it were not for the rapid closure (inactivation) of the Na^+-channels
- At the same time there is a constant background movement of K^+ out of the cell. This has the effect of placing a limit on the change of membrane potential during the depolarisation phase of the action potential
- During repolarisation, there is the opening of the voltage-sensitive K^+-channels, leading to loss

of K^+ from the cell. These react more slowly than the Na^+-channels, and are open for longer. Thus, repolarisation, with a return to the resting membrane potential is a slower process than depolarisation

- After lots of action potentials, when there is the exchange of many ions, the ionic environment is returned to the steady state by the continued and persistent action of the Na^+/K^+ pumps

7. What is meant by the 'refractory period'?

This is the temporary state immediately after an action potential when no further action potentials may be initiated. It can be divided into:

- *Absolute refractory period:* the first stage of this phase when no action potentials may be generated, irrespective of the amplitude of the stimulus
- *Relative refractory period:* the latter part of this phase, when the cell membrane may be brought to threshold only with a larger-than-normal stimulus

8. What is the effect of myelination on a nerve fibre?

Myelinated fibres have their axons enveloped with the myelin and cell bodies of a Schwann cell (or oligodendrocyte in the CNS). This has a number of effects on propagation of action potentials along the axons of the myelinated neurones, compared to unmyelinated ones:

- *The conduction velocity is increased:* the larger fibres of the myelinated neurone have lower resistance to current flow due to a larger number of intracellular ions
- *Saltatory conduction:* current is generated at the nodes of Ranvier only, and not at the myelin sheath. Consequently, the current *jumps* quickly between nodes, reducing the time for the delivery of signals

ACTION POTENTIALS

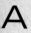

9. What types of nerve fibres are there?

Peripheral nerve fibres may be classified in the following way:

- *Group A:* These are the largest (up to 20 μm):
  - α (Ia and Ib): Motor and proprioception fibres
  - β (II): Touch, pressure and proprioception fibres
  - γ (II): Muscle spindle fusimotor fibres
  - δ (III): Touch pain and pressure fibres
- *Group B:* Myelinated fibres which are autonomic preganglionic (up to 3 μm)
- *Group C (type IV):* Unmyelinated fibres which carry postganglionic fibres, and fibres for touch and pain (up to 2 μm)

10. Briefly list some drugs that may alter the conduction along a neurone.

Some agents which can modify the activation and propagation of the action potential include:

- *Tetrodotoxin:* a neurotoxin that is a selective blocker of Na^+-channels
- *Tetraethylammonium:* a selective K^+-channel blocker, which prolongs the action potential
- *Local anaesthetic agents:* composed of an amine group connected to an aromatic side chain via an ester or amide bond. They are selective blockers of the voltage-dependent Na^+-channels

ADRENAL CORTEX I

1. What are the anatomic layers of the adrenal cortex, and which hormones do they produce?

- *Zona glomerulosa:* the superficial layer. Mineralocorticoid production occurs here
- *Zona fasiculata:* the middle layer
- *Zona reticularis:* the deepest layer
- The deepest two layers are for the production of glucocorticoids, androgens, and oestrogens. Progestogens are also produced, but they act mainly as precursors in the production of the other hormones

2. What is the basic composition of these hormones?

They are all steroid hormones, with a common cyclo-pentanoperhydrophenanthrene ring structure at the core of the molecule.

3. From which molecule are these hormones all derived?

The common source is dietary cholesterol. This is converted to another precursor, pregnenolone by enzymes of the cytochrome P450 system.

4. What are the main mineralocorticoids, glucocorticoids, androgens and oestrogens produced?

- *Mineralocorticoid:* Aldosterone
- *Glucocorticoid:* Cortisol
- *Androgen:* Dehydroepiandrosterone (DHEA)
- *Oestrogen:* Oestradiol. Only a small amount of this is secreted

5. What are the physiological effects of aldosterone?

- *Sodium balance:* stimulation of sodium reabsorption in the distal convoluted tubule (DCT) and collecting duct of the kidney, sweat glands, salivary glands and gut

- *Potassium balance:* through the active exchange with sodium ions at the membrane, leading to the loss of serum potassium

- *Acid-Base balance:* H^+ may also be exchanged with Na^+, leading to loss of H^+ from the plasma. Therefore, aldosterone excess may lead to a metabolic alkalosis

- *Water balance:* as a consequence of increasing the serum $[Na^+]$, there is stimulation of pituitary osmoreceptors, leading to increased release of arginine vasopressin (AVP) (also known as antidiuretic hormone (ADH)). This leads to water retention, and so a return of the $[Na^+]$ back to normal at the expense of increased circulating volume

6. Describe the principle mechanisms controlling aldosterone release

Aldosterone release is stimulated by

- *Increased renin secretion:* this increases the serum aldosterone through increasing serum angiotensin II. Important stimuli for the release of renin is reduction of renal perfusion and reduced presentation of sodium to the kidney's macula densa
- *Decrease of plasma* $[Na^+]$
- *Increase of plasma* $[K^+]$

Aldosterone secretion is reduced by the opposite of the above together with

- *Increased circulating atrial natriuretic peptide (ANP):* this has an inhibitory effect on renin release, and so acts indirectly to inhibit aldosterone release

7. Where is renin produced?

In the kidney, from the cells of the juxtaglomerular apparatus.

8. Summarise the main effects of glucocorticoids.

- *Metabolic effects* (see below)
- *Mineralocorticoid actions:* lead to stimulation of sodium and water retention, together with the loss of potassium
- *Anti-inflammatory effects*
- *Immunosuppressive actions*
- *Control of the body's stress response*
- *Others:* e.g. antagonism of the effects of vitamin D_3 metabolites on calcium balance and various effects on circulating blood cells

9. What are the principle metabolic effects?

These involve changes in the metabolism of carbohydrates, fats and proteins

- *Carbohydrate:* has a hyperglycaemic effect. Antagonises the effects of insulin, and stimulates gluconeogenesis
- *Protein:* stimulates amino acid uptake and protein synthesis in the liver, while inhibiting uptake in the peripheral tissues. In large quantities, leads to muscle wasting following increased peripheral protein mobilisation
- *Fats:* stimulates lipolysis at physiological levels of secretion

10. What is the basic mechanism of action of the adrenal cortical hormones?

In common with all steroid hormones, they all act through intracellular receptor binding leading to gene stimulation. They are lipophillic, and so are able to penetrate the cytoplasm and nuclear envelope easily.

ADRENAL CORTEX II – CLINICAL DISORDERS

1. What types of hyperaldosteronism are there, and what basic features characterise each?

- *Primary hyperaldosteronism:* or Conn's syndrome, due to autonomous secretion by the adrenal cortex
- *Secondary:* associated with increased levels of hormones of the renin-angiotensin-aldosterone (R-A-A) system, e.g. following dehydration, blood loss, cardiac and liver failure with third-spacing of fluid. Also occurs with renal artery stenosis

2. What causes Conn's syndrome?

It is most often due to a single (rarely more) adenoma of the zona glomerulosa of the adrenal cortex. Also following idiopathic bilateral hyperplasia of the zona glomerulosa.

3. What is the dominant clinical feature?

Hypertension due to chronic salt and water retention. Peripheral odema is not, however, usually present despite water excess – the mechanism for this is not understood fully.

4. What biochemical abnormalities might you detect?

- *Hypernatraemia:* following salt retention. However, water retention may lead to a normal plasma [Na$^+$]
- *Hypokalaemia:* patients may have associated muscle weakness and cardiac arrhythmias
- *Metabolic alkalosis:* associated with hypokalaemia and loss of H$^+$ following increased exchange with Na$^+$ at the kidney

5. What will the urine show?
- Increased potassium
- Low sodium
- High aldosterone concentrations

6. Apart from the important features mentioned above, what other clinical feature commonly occurs with Conn's syndrome?

Polyuria. This is due to tubular nephropathy, leading to a reversible diabetes insipidus.

7. Which aldosterone antagonist has been used in the medical management of this disorder?

The diuretic *spironalactone*.

8. What are the most common causes of Cushing's syndrome of cortisol excess?

In their order of frequency:
- *Iatrogenic steroid administration*
- *Cushing's disease:* due to an adenoma of the pituitary leading to over secretion of adrenocorticotrophic hormone (ACTH)
- *Ectopic ACTH secretion:* such as a peripheral tumour, often in the lung
- *Adrenal adenoma:* leading to hypersecretion of cortisol. Note that unlike the above two cases, cortisol excess here is autonomous and independent of ACTH
- *Adrenal carcinoma*

9. What clinical features might you find on examination of a patient with Cushing's syndrome?
- *General features:* central fat distribution with a 'bull-hump'. Associated peripheral muscle wasting. Presence of a plethoric, 'moon-face', hirsutism

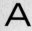

- *Skin:* may show bruises and poor wound healing and atrophy. Also abdominal striae
- *Spine:* may show kyphosis due to osteoporotic collapse of vertebrae
- *Bi-temporal hemianopia:* due to a pituitary tumour compressing the optic chiasm
- *Hypertension*
- *Urine dipstick shows glucosuria*

10. What are the principle causes of adrenal insufficiency?

- *Auto-immune adrenalitis:* leading to Addison's disease
- *TB:* of the adrenal glands
- Less commonly due to tumours, amyloid or other bacterial infection of the glands

11. What is the most common cause of congenital adrenal hyperplasia?

21-hydroxylase deficiency. This leads to ACTH excess following reduced glucocorticoid and mineralocorticoid synthesis. Can produce congenital hyperkalaemia and an Addisonian crisis with vomiting and dehydration. Since the path of hormone production goes down that of androgen synthesis, leads to developmentally ambiguous genitalia.

ADRENAL MEDULLA

1. How does the embryonic origin of the adrenal cortex differ from that of the medulla?

The adrenal cortex is mesodermal in origin, whereas the medulla is derived from neuroectoderm. This determines the pattern of innervation of the adrenal gland.

2. What are the two major hormones produced by the adrenal medulla? What is the ratio of production for each?

The catecholamines
- Epinephrine (80% of output)
- Norepinephrine (20% of output)
- However, there are many others produced to a lesser degree by the chromaffin cells, such as dopamine, somatostatin, substance P and enkephalins

3. What is the precursor for these hormones?

Tyrosine: this amino acid may itself be formed from another amino acid, *phenylalanine*.

4. Briefly describe the path of production, including the names of the enzymes at each step.

Catecholamine synthesis may be summarised in the following flow chart:

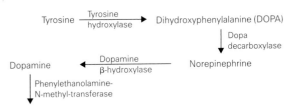

Reprinted by permission of Oxford University Press from Laycock, Wise. Essential Endocrinology 3rd, 1996

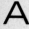

5. How is the adrenal medulla innervated?

Preganglionic sympathetic fibres synapse directly onto the chromaffin cells of the adrenal medulla. As with other preganglionic autonomic synapses, the neuro-transmitter at this point is *acetylcholine (ACh)*.

ACh release from the preganglionic sympathetic fibre stimulates the release of catecholamines by exocytosis, just in the same manner as any other synapse.

Therefore, in effect, the chromaffin cells are specialised postganglionic sympathetic neurones that secrete their transmitter directly into the circulation. The origin of this arrangement arises from the neuroectodermal origin of the adrenal medulla.

6. What are the metabolic effects of sympathetic stimulation by the catecholamines?

The metabolic effects are mainly on carbohydrate and lipid homeostasis:

- *Carbohydrate:* catecholamines cause hyperglycaemia. Epinephrine stimulates hepatic gluconeogenesis and glycogenolysis. Also, both epinephrine and norepinephrine inhibit the release of insulin from β-islet cells of the pancreas. This is mediated through *α-adrenoceptors*
- *Lipid:* epinephrine (and to a smaller extent norepinephrine) stimulates lipolysis in adipose tissue, which increases the plasma free fatty acid (FFA) concentration
- Note that the catecholamines also cause a general increase in the basal metabolic rate (BMR)

7. How are these hormones metabolised?

This can be summarised as a flow diagram:

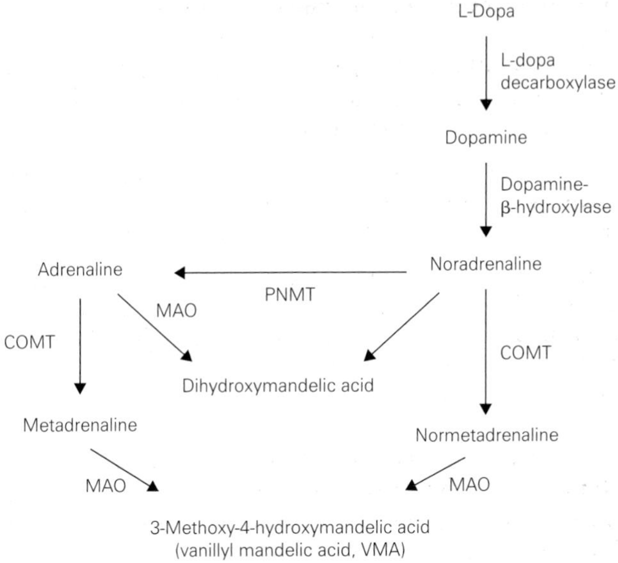

A

L-Dopa

↓ L-dopa decarboxylase

Dopamine

↓ Dopamine-β-hydroxylase

Adrenaline ← PNMT ← Noradrenaline

MAO

COMT

Dihydroxymandelic acid

Metadrenaline

COMT

Normetadrenaline

MAO → ← MAO

3-Methoxy-4-hydroxymandelic acid
(vanillyl mandelic acid, VMA)

Metabolism of Catecholamines
Where COMT = Catechol-O-methyl transferase, MAO = Monoamine oxidase
Reprinted by permission of Oxford University Press from Laycock, Wise.
Essential Endocrinology 3rd, 1996

ADRENAL MEDULLA

8. What are the physiological effects of phaeochromocytoma?

This can be thought of as a syndrome of paroxysmal, intermittent, but generalised sympathetic stimulation leading to:

- *Cardiovascular effects*:
  - Hypertensive episodes that may be severe enough to lead to stroke, myocardial infarction (MI), etc.
  - Tachycardia and palpitations
  - Pallor
- *Gastrointestinal:* diarrhoea
- *Metabolic:* hyperglycaemia and glucose intolerance

9. What biochemical tests may be performed to make the diagnosis?

A number of tests can be performed to establish the diagnosis, predominantly based on measuring catecholamine metabolites:

- 24 urinary measurement of *vanillyl mandelic acid:* the traditional investigation, but misses 30% of cases of phaeochromocytoma
- Metadrenaline: more sensitive than the above
- Plasma or urinary epinephrine or norepinephrine: best measured during hypertensive episodes

10. Which drug is used in the management of this condition?

Phenoxybenzamine: this is an α-adrenoceptor antagonist.

11. How are the multiple endocrine neoplasia (MEN) syndromes classified?

These conditions essentially occur in three groups:

- *Type I:* adenomas of the parathyroid, pancreatic and anterior pituitary glands
- *Type IIa:* hyperparathyroidism, phaeochromocytoma, medullary carcinoma of the thyroid
- *Type IIb:* phaeochromocytoma, medullary carcinoma of the thyroid, with multiple cutaneous neuromas and neurofibromas

ARTERIAL PRESSURE

A

1. Draw the arterial pressure waveform, and label the axes.

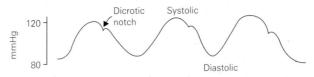

Arterial pressure waveform

The 'dicrotic notch' is a momentary rise in the arterial pressure trace following closure of the aortic valve.

2. How is the mean arterial pressure (MAP) calculated from this waveform?

This is calculated by dividing the area under the pressure wave by the time measured.

3. How may the MAP be calculated simply?

By the formula:

Diastolic pressure +
1/3 (systolic pressure − diastolic pressure)

4. Why is the mean pressure not a simple average of the systolic and diastolic pressures?

This is because the mean pressure is time-weighted, and for about 2/3 of the time cycle, the pressure is close to the diastolic level.

5. What is blood pressure?

This is defined as the product of the CO and the SVR.

A

6. How does the arterial pressure waveform differ at the aortic root compared to further distally in the arterial tree? Why does this occur?

These differences are in part, due to changes in wall stiffness along the arterial tree, and its consequent effects on the transmission of the pulse wave along the vessel

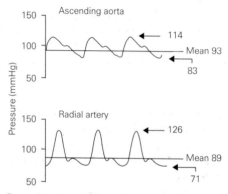

Pressure waves at different sites in the arterial tree. With transmission of the pressure wave into the distal aorta and large arteries, the systolic pressure increases and the diastolic pressure decreases, with a resultant heightening of the pulse pressure. However, the mean arterial pressure declines steadily.

Adapted from Smith & Kampire. Circulatory Physiology, 3rd edition, 1990, Lippincott, Williams & Wilkins

7. What are the two basic mechanisms involved in the control of the arterial pressure?

- *Short-term regulation:* by neuronal pathways involving a multineuronal reflex arc consisting of receptors, afferent pathways, and effectors
- *Long-term regulation:* by the control of the extracellular fluid (ECF) volume. This is especially important after a period of fluid depletion

AUTONOMIC NERVOUS SYSTEM (ANS)

A

1. What are the components of the ANS?

The sympathetic and parasympathetic nervous systems (SNS and PNS).

2. Where are the locations of the cell bodies of the neurones that make up the SNS?

- *Preganglionic cells:* cell bodies are located at the lateral horns of the spinal grey matter. This extends from T1 to L2 *(thoraco-lumbar outflow)*
- *Postganglionic cells:* cell bodies are located in the sympathetic chain

3. Other than their location, how else do pre and postganglionic cells of the SNS differ?

- *Preganglionic fibres are myelinated:* therefore, their diameter is larger with more rapid transmission of the action potential
- *Differences in the neurotransmitter:* the transmitter substance secreted by preganglionic cells is ACh (acting on nicotinic receptors), and by postganglionic cells is *noradrenaline*

4. What is special about the mode of sympathetic supply to the adrenal medulla?

The chromaffin cells of the adrenal medulla receive direct innervation from preganglionic sympathetic fibres arising from the lateral horn of the spinal cord. Stimulation leads to secretion of catacholamine from the chromaffin cells, so these cells are akin to postganglionic cells of the SNS.

5. How does the origin of the PNS differ from the SNS?

- *Preganglionic parasympathetic:* these neurones take origin from specific cranial nerve nuclei and from sacral segments 2–4 of the spinal cord *(cranio-sacral outflow vs. thoraco-lumbar origin of the SNS)*
- *Parasympathetic ganglia:* unlike the sympathetic chain, the PNS ganglia are located at discrete points close to their respective target organs

6. Which cranial nerves have a parasympathetic outflow?

Cranial nerves III, VII, IX and X.

7. Taking all of this into account, summarise briefly the neurotransmitters of the ANS, and which types of receptor they act on.

- *Preganglionic cells:* the cells of both systems release ACh at the synapse with the postganglionic cells. It acts on *nicotinic* cholinoceptors
- *Postganglionic cells:* PNS – ACh is released, acting on muscarinic cholinoceptors. SNS – *noradrenaline* acting on α- or *β-adrenoceptors*

8. Generally speaking, how does the distribution of parasympathetic innervation in the body differ from sympathetic distribution?

- *Parasympathetic fibres are visceral:* they do not supply the trunk or limbs
- *Parasympathetic fibres do not supply the gonads or adrenal glands*

9. Which second messengers are important for the function of the different types of receptors in the ANS?

The most important second messengers through which the cholinoceptors and adrenoceptors function are cyclic adenosine monophosphate (cAMP), diacylglycerol (DAG) and inositol diphosphate (IP_2).

- α_1-*adrenoceptors:* stimulation causes an increase of intracellular *phospholipase C,* leading to an increase of the second messengers IP_2 and DAG. This causes activation of a number of protein kinases, and stimulates release of intracellular Ca^{2+} stores. (So, in the cases of arterioles, leads to vasoconstriction following stimulation of mural smooth muscle contraction)

- α_2-*adrenoceptors:* stimulation leads to *inhibition* of the enzyme adenylyl cyclase, reducing the intracellular levels of the second messenger cAMP

- β_1 *and* β_2-*adrenoceptors:* act through *stimulation* of adenylyl cyclase, leading to increases of intracellular cAMP. This goes on to activate a number of protein kinases important in producing the desired effect on the target organ

- *Muscarinic cholinoceptors:* although these are G-protein coupled receptors, the exact system of second-messenger signalling has not been fully elucidated

- *Nicotinic cholinoceptors:* these are not G-protein coupled, but are directly linked to ion channels

10. Give some examples of the results of stimulation of the various adrenoceptors by noradrenaline.

The effects may be summarised by the following table:

Effects mediated by adrenoceptor subtypes

A

AUTONOMIC NERVOUS SYSTEM

	Adrenoceptor			
Tissue	α_1	α_2	β_1	β_2
Smooth muscle				
Blood vessels	Constrict	Constrict		Dilate
Bronchi	Constrict			Dilate
GI tract				
Non-sphincter	Relax (hyperpolarisation)		Relax (no hyperpolarisation)	
Sphincter	Contract			
Uterus	Contract			Relax
Bladder				
Detrusor				Relax
Sphincter	Contract			
Seminal tract	Contract			Relax
Iris (radial)	Contract			
Ciliary muscle				Relax
Heart			Incr rate Incr force	
Skeletal muscle				Tremor
Liver	Glycogenolysis K⁺ release			Glycogenolysis
Fat			Lipolysis	
Nerve terminals				
Adrenergic		Decr release	Incr release	
Cholinergic (some)		Decr release		
Salivary gland	K⁺ release		Amylase secretion	
Platelets		Aggregation		
Mast cells				Inhibition of histamine release
Second messengers	IP₃, DAG	↓cAMP	↑cAMP	↑cAMP

CARBON DIOXIDE TRANSPORT

1. In which forms is CO_2 transported in the blood?

There are three ways:

- *As the bicarbonate ion (HCO_3^-):* accounts for 85–90% of carriage
- *As carbamino compounds:* formed when CO_2 binds with the terminal amine group of plasma proteins. 5–10% of CO_2 is transported in this way
- *Physically dissolved in solution:* accounts for 5%

2. How does the mode of CO_2 transport differ between arterial and venous blood?

In arterial blood, there is *less* carbamino compound carriage and *more* bicarbonate carriage. The amount physically dissolved varies little between the two circulations. The variation is due to the difference in pH affecting the binding and dissociation properties of the molecule.

3. How does the amount of CO_2 physically dissolved in the plasma compare to the amount of dissolved oxygen?

Only about 1% of the oxygen in the blood is dissolved in the plasma. This is because CO_2 is some 24 times more water-soluble than oxygen.

4. You mentioned that CO_2 combines with plasma proteins to form carbamino compounds. What is the most significant of these plasma proteins?

Haemoglobin. CO_2 binds to its globin chain.

5. How does CO_2 come to be carried as the bicarbonate ion?

Through the reaction:

$$CO_2 + H_2O \rightleftharpoons H_2CO_3 \rightleftharpoons H^+ + HCO_3^-$$

This reaction is catalysed by the enzyme *carbonic anhydrase*.

6. What happens to all of the H⁺ generated by this process?

This is 'mopped-up' by other buffer systems. This is of particular importance in the red cell, where the H^+ generated cannot escape due to cell membrane impermeability. In this case, the H^+ binds with (i.e. is buffered by) the haemoglobin molecule (mainly the imidazole groups of the polypeptide chain).

7. What effect does all of this haemoglobin-binding of H⁺ have on the transport of oxygen by this molecule?

The addition of H^+ and CO_2 to the haemoglobin chain leads to a reduced oxygen affinity. This is seen as a *right shift* in the oxygen dissociation curve.

8. What is the fate of all the bicarbonate generated in the red blood cell when it carries CO₂?

The bicarbonate formed diffuses out of the red cell and into the plasma (unlike H^+, it is able to penetrate the red cell membrane). To maintain electrochemical neutrality, a Cl^- ion enters the red cell at the same time as the bicarbonate leaves. This is known as the *chloride shift*.

9. How does the transport of CO₂ affect the osmotic balance of the red cell?

All of the bicarbonate and Cl^- generated following CO_2 carriage by the red cell increases the intracellular osmotic pressure. This causes the cell to swell with extra H_2O that diffuses through the cell membrane. This is why the haematocrit (HCT) of venous blood is some 3% higher than in arterial blood.

▼

10. How does the shape of the oxygen dissociation curve differ from the CO_2 dissociation curve? Show this by drawing graphs.

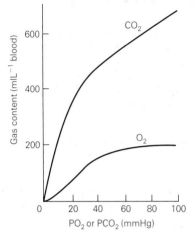

From Lecture Notes on Human Physiology, 3rd edition, Bray, Cragg, Macknight, Mills & Taylor, 1994, Oxford, Blackwell Science

- The CO_2 dissociation curve is *curvi-linear*
- The O_2 dissociation curve is *sigmoidal*

11. Why cannot the amount of CO_2 in the blood be expressed as a *percent-saturation*, unlike the case for oxygen?

Since CO_2 is so much more water-soluble than O_2, it never reaches saturation point. Therefore, its blood saturation cannot reasonably be expressed as a percentage of a total level. This can be seen in the CO_2 dissociation curve – it never reaches a peak, but continues to rise in linear fashion.

12. What is the difference between the *Bohr* effect and the *Haldane* effect?

- The *Bohr* effect describes the changes in the affinity of the haemoglobin chain for oxygen following variations in the $PaCO_2$, H^+ and temperature

- The *Haldane* describes changes in the affinity of the blood for CO_2 with variations in the PaO_2. As the PaO_2 *increases*, the affinity of the blood for CO_2 *decreases*, seen as a *downward* shift in the CO_2 dissociation curve

CARDIAC CYCLE

1. What is the duration of the cardiac cycle at rest?

0.8–0.9 s.

2. Below is a diagram of the pressure changes in the left side of the heart during the cardiac cycle. What do the points A, B, C, and D represent?

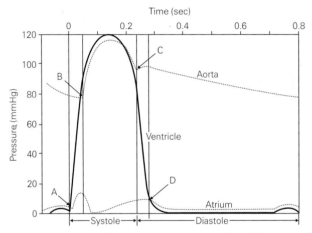

From Smith & Kampire. Circulatory Physiology, 3rd edition, 1990, Lippincott, Williams & Wilkins

- A: closure of the mitral valve at the onset of ventricular systole
- B: opening of the aortic valve at the onset of rapid ventricular ejection
- C: closure of the aortic valve, forming the 'dicrotic notch'
- D: opening of the mitral valve and ventricular filling at the onset of ventricular diastole

3. What name is given to the portion of the cycle between A and B? What is its significance?

This is the stage of *isovolumetric contraction*. During this stage, both the AV valves and arterial valves are closed, so that the ventricle is a closed chamber. The onset of contraction causes a rapid rise in the wall tension at constant volume. The rapidity of the rise of this tension (dP/dt) is used as a measure of the myocardial contractility.

4. Define the stroke volume. Give a typical value for this and the ejection fraction.

This is defined as the volume ejected by the ventricles during ventricular systole, and is equal to the difference between the end-diastolic and end-systolic volumes.

Typically it is $120 - 40 = 80$ ml. The ejection fraction is about 0.67.

5. What is the name given to the point in the cycle between B and C? How does it relate to the aortic root pressure?

This is the phase of rapid ventricular ejection. It is heralded by the opening of the arterial valves, when the ventricular pressure exceeds the pressure at the root of the aorta and pulmonary trunk.

Normally, there is little pressure difference between the root of the aorta and the left ventricle during this phase. Therefore, the pressure profiles of both are closely matched with the ventricular pressure being only slightly higher.

6. What causes the dicrotic notch in the aortic root pressure at the end of rapid ventricular ejection?

This is the consequence of the reversed pressure gradient occurring at the aortic root towards the end of systole. The outward momentum generated across the aortic valve following rapid ejection ensures continued

▼

flow, despite a higher pressure in the aortic root. When the valve does finally close, it does so forcefully, causing the brief pressure rise known as the dicrotic notch.

7. Why is there a small rise in the atrial pressure just before the onset of ventricular systole?

This pressure rise is due to the atrial 'kick'. Ventricular filling is predominantly a passive process occurring when the atrial pressure exceeds the ventricular pressure during diastole. The final atrial 'kick' is the only active part of this process when the atrium contracts. At rest, it contributes to about 20% of final ventricular filling.

8. Draw the diagram of the electrocardiogram (ECG) waveform and the timing of the heart sounds.

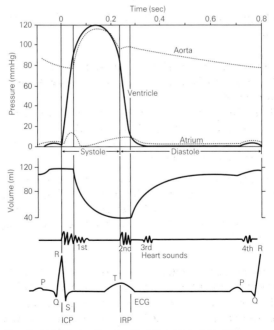

From Smith & Kampire. Circulatory Physiology, 3rd edition, 1990, Lippincott, Williams & Wilkins

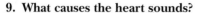

C

9. What causes the heart sounds?

- *First sound:* closure of the AV valves
- *Second sound:* closure of the arterial valves
- *Third sound:* due to rapid ventricular filling, and heard after the second sound. It is often a normal phenomenon in the young
- *Fourth sound:* associated with cardiac disease, being caused by rapid atrial contraction filling a stiff ventricle. It is heard before the first heart sound

10. Briefly describe the effect of exercise on the phase duration of the cardiac cycle.

During exercise, all of the phases of the cycle shorten, but ventricular diastole becomes disproportionably shorter, with a marked reduction of the diastolic filling time. (During rest, diastole accounts for about 2/3 of the cardiac cycle.)

To offset the reduction in the diastolic filling time, the atrial 'kick' at the end of ventricular diastole contributes more to ventricular filling. Thus, if the heart rate were increased in isolation, the CO would actually fall since there is a marked reduction in end-diastolic volume that occurs with shorter diastolic filling.

CARDIAC OUTPUT (CO)

1. What is the definition of the CO?

This is defined as the product of the heart rate and the stroke volume.

2. Give a normal resting value for the CO.

$5–6\,Lmin^{-1}$.

3. How do the outputs of the two ventricles compare to one another?

In the normal state, the outputs of both ventricles are essentially equal – both being $5–6\,Lmin^{-1}$.

4. Which factors influence the stroke volume?

- Preload
- Afterload
- Myocardial contractility
- Heart rate

5. What determines the preload?

This is determined by the venous return to the heart. The amount of venous return itself depends on the difference between the systemic filling pressure (driving blood back to the heart) and the central venous pressure (CVP) (working against the venous return).

CARDIAC OUTPUT

C

6. Define the afterload. What is this analogous to, in simple terms?

This is the ventricular wall tension that has to be generated in order to eject blood out of the ventricle. It is analogous to the arterial pressure. An increase in the CO causes a rise in the arterial pressure (afterload). This in turn, has a negative feedback effect on the output. Since more energy is consumed generating a high enough pressure to overcome a high arterial pressure, the resulting stroke volume is less – reducing the output in subsequent beats.

7. What happens to the Frank-Starling curve of the heart when the myocardial contractility is increased?

There is an upwards shift of the curve, so that the stroke volume is higher for any given end diastolic volume.

8. What causes a rise in the myocardial contractility?

- *Intrinsic:* direct stimulation of cardiac sympathetic fibres by the ANS
- *Extrinsic:* stimulation of myocardial β_1-adrenoceptors by circulating catacholamines

9. Aside from increasing the myocardial contractility, by what other mechanisms does sympathetic stimulation increase the CO?

- There is an increase in the heart rate
- It stimulates peripheral venoconstriction, which increases the venous return to the heart, and through the Frank-Starling mechanism increases the stroke volume

Note that the CO is therefore determined by the interplay of a number of related factors. These relationships may be summarised by the following flow diagram:

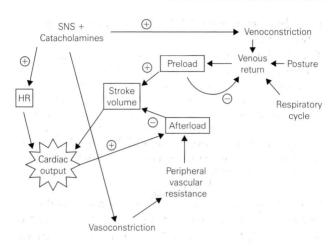

CELL SIGNALLING

1. Which parts of a cell express receptors?

Receptors may be located at the cell membrane, or within the cytosol of the cell.

2. Can you name the four main types of receptor involved in cellular signalling? Give some examples.

- *Ion channel linked receptor:* e.g. nicotinic cholinoceptors at the neuromuscular junction
- *G-protein coupled receptor:* e.g. muscarinic cholinoceptors and adrenoceptors
- *Tyrosine kinase linked receptor:* e.g. various growth factors, insulin receptor
- *Intracellular receptor:* steroid hormone receptors

3. What basically happens when a ligand binds to a G-protein coupled receptor?

Receptor stimulation by the ligand causes binding of the receptor to its G-protein. This causes the G-protein to release (inactive) guanosine diphosphate (GDP) and uptake (active) guanosine triphosphate (GTP). Depending on the type of G-protein that the receptor is coupled to, the G-protein may then activate the enzyme adenylyl cyclase, or inhibit it, or it may stimulate the enzyme phospholipase C.

4. What are the components of the G-protein?

This is composed of α, β and γ subunits:

- α subunit: variation in this determines the type of G-protein. This component binds to GDP and GTP
- β and γ components bind reversibly to the α subunit

5. What is the functional significance of the α subunit?

This determines the type of G-protein and therefore its function. There are several types of α subunit, each linked to a particular type of G-protein. Three examples are:

- G_s: receptor binding to this system leads to activation of adenylyl cyclase, e.g. occurs with β_1- and β_2-adrenoceptor stimulation and glucagon signals through this pathway
- G_i: receptor binding to this system leads to inhibition of adenylyl cyclase, e.g. with α_2-adrenoceptor stimulation
- G_q: binding produces activation of phospholipase C, e.g. α_1-adrenoceptors

6. What is the result of activation or inhibition of adenylyl cyclase by the activated G-protein?

This leads to an increase or decrease in intracellular *cAMP*, respectively. This molecule is termed a *second messenger*, since it is an intermediary product following G-protein coupled receptor stimulation. It stimulates molecules within the cell, such as protein kinases, leading to activation of many intracellular reaction cascades.

7. Can you give some more examples of other second messengers generated through G-protein receptor stimulation? What effects do these have within the cell?

- *DAG:* this is produced when activated phospholipase C (generated from G_q-protein linked receptor stimulation) hydrolyses inositol triphosphate (IP_3). DAG stimulates various cellular protein kinases
- *IP_2:* this is also generated by hydrolysis of IP_3 by activated phospholipase C. IP_2 has the effect of causing Ca^{2+} release from the endoplasmic reticulum, such as occurs during activation of smooth muscle cells
- *Cyclic guanosine monophosphate (cGMP):* leads to activation of protein kinase G
- *Arachidonic acid and eicosanoids:* these are produced by G-protein linked receptors that activate

phospholipase A_2. These have numerous effects following production of prostaglandins

8. Do G-protein coupled receptors always produce their effects through second messenger pathways?

No, in some instances, these receptors are linked directly to ion channels, such as some types of K^+-channel.

9. What is the single most important effect of stimulation of any kind of tyrosine kinase linked receptor?

Mitogenesis: This type of receptor is important in the stimulation of cellular growth and division. In keeping with this, it is the method of signalling for insulin and a number of growth factors – such as *epidermal growth factor* (EGF) and *platelet-derived growth factor* (PDGF). In this respect, a number of oncogenes encode for portions of tyrosine kinase receptors.

10. What is the basic structure of the tyrosine kinase linked receptor?

This is a transmembrane enzyme composed of a number of subunits that have specific functions determined by their position in relation to the cell membrane.

11. What is so distinctive about the way that it signals?

Following ligand binding, the receptor phosphorylates itself (*autophosphorylation*). Following this phenomenon, the receptor further phosphorylates target intracellular proteins with greater efficiency.

12. Generally speaking, what kinds of hormones signal directly through intracellular receptors? Give examples.

Lipophilic molecules that are able to penetrate the lipid bilayer of the cell membrane. Important examples are the steroid hormones (glucocorticoids and

C

mineralocorticoids of the adrenal cortex, gonadal hormones) and the thyroid hormones.

13. How do these produce their effects?

The lipophilic hormone crosses the cell membrane and binds to the intracellular receptor. The complex formed then translocates to the nucleus of the cell through the nuclear envelope. By binding onto the DNA of the cell, this complex stimulates directly the transcription of specific genes for protein production.

14. How does the duration of action of this form of cell signalling differ from other types?

Hormones that signal through intracellular receptors generally have a longer duration of action than hormones that signal through other means. This is because of the complex cascade of reactions stimulated. It also follows that they also have a slower onset of activity since proteins have to be synthesised before the final actions can occur.

CELL SIGNALLING

C CEREBROSPINAL FLUID (CSF) AND CEREBRAL BLOOD FLOW

1. What is the volume of the CSF?

150 ml. It is produced at a rate of ~500 ml per day.

2. Where is it produced?

- *Choroid plexus:* of the intracerebral ventricles. Accounts for 70% of production
- *Blood vessels lining ventricular walls:* accounts for 30% of production

3. Briefly describe the CSF circulation.

- From the lateral ventricle, the CSF flows into the 3rd ventricles by way of the interventricular foramen of Monro
- From the 3rd ventricles, it flows into the 4th through the aqueduct of Sylvius
- Some of the CSF now passes into the central canal of the spinal cord as a continuation of the 4th ventricle
- The majority flows from the 4th ventricle into the sub-arachnoid space of the spinal cord through the central foramen of Magendie and the two laterally placed foramina of Luschka
- After going around the spinal cord, it enters the cranial cavity through the foramen magnum, and flows around the sub-arachnoid space of the brain

4. Where is the CSF finally absorbed?

- *The arachnoid villi:* accounts for 80% of absorption
- *Spinal nerve roots:* accounts for 20% of absorption

5. What are the arachnoid villi composed of?

These are formed from the fusion of arachnoid membrane and the endothelium of a dural venous sinus that it bulges into.

6. What is the rate of cerebral blood flow?

50 ml per 100 g of brain tissue. It accounts for 15% of the CO, or about 750 mlmin^{-1}.

7. How does this rate of flow vary with the arterial pressure?

The rate of flow remains essentially stable owing to local autoregulation of flow. This is a characteristic feature of some specialised vascular beds, such as the renal system.

8. What is the basic mechanism of autoregulation?

There are two principle reasons:

- *Myogenic response:* an increase in the arteriolar wall tension brought on by an increase in the arterial pressure stimulates contraction of the mural smooth muscle cells. The resulting vasoconstriction stabilises the flow in the face of these pressure changes

- *Vasodilator 'washout':* if flow is suddenly and momentarily increased by a sudden rise in the driving pressure, locally-produced vasodilating mediators are washed out of the vessel, leading to vasoconstriction and a return of the flow to the steady state

9. What are the main factors that govern the cerebral blood flow?

- *$PaCO_2$:* hypercarbia increases the cerebral flow through an increase of the $[H^+]$. The reverse occurs with hypocarbia

- *PaO_2:* hypoxia produces cerebral vasodilatation, increasing the flow. This influence is less important than the above

- *Sympathetic stimulation:* causes some vasoconstriction, but this is the least important influence

10. What is meant by the cerebral perfusion pressure?

This is defined as the difference between the mean arterial pressure and the intracranial pressure. It must remain above around 70 mmHg for adequate cerebral perfusion.

COLON

C

1. What are the major functions of the colon?

- *Absorption of water:* the most important
- *Absorption of minerals:* predominantly sodium. There is, however, net secretion of potassium and bicarbonate
- *Expulsion of faeces*
- *Indirect role:* bacterial flora in the colon are able to synthesise vitamin K and some of the B vitamins. They also produce some important fatty acids

2. What types of contraction does the colon have in common with the small bowel?

- *Segmentation:* this mixes the contents of the colon, facilitating absorption
- *Peristalsis:* propelling the contents distally

COLON

3. What type of contraction is peculiar to the colon?

Mass action contraction. There is simultaneous contraction of the smooth muscle over a very long length. This moves material from one portion of the colon to another in one movement. It occurs between 1–3 times per day.

4. Identify one way in which the basic electric rhythm of the colon differs from that of the small bowel.

Unlike in the small bowel, the frequency of the wave of contraction increases along the colon. At the ileocaecal valve it is 2 per minute, and in the sigmoid colon, up to 6 per minute.

5. What is the *gastro-colic* reflex?

This occurs after a meal enters the stomach, leading to an increase in the motility of the proximal and distal

▼

C

colon, together with an increase in the frequency of
mass movements.

6. Outline the events that occur during defecation.

- The defecation reflex is triggered by the distension
  of the rectal walls by faeces entering from a mass
  contraction proximally
- The intra-rectal pressure has to reach 18 mmHg
  before the reflex is triggered
- Afferent impulses pass to sacral segments 2, 3 and 4.
  This leads to stimulation of the efferent reflex
  pathway, together with stimulation of the thalamus
  and cortical sensory areas producing the conscious
  desire to defecate
- Efferent impulses pass back to the myenteric plexus
  of the rectum, activating postganglionic PNS
  neurones
- This leads to contraction, propelling the faeces
  forward
- PNS stimulation also leads to *relaxation* of the
  internal anal sphincter
- The external sphincter relaxes, reducing the
  pressure in the anal canal. Further peristalsis in the
  rectum pushes the faeces out
- This is augmented by voluntary contractions of the
  pelvic floor muscles when performing the Valsalva
  manoeuvre

7. What happens to the reflex pathway when there is conscious desire not to defecate?

When faecal material enters the upper anal canal, there
is stimulation of S1, 2 and 3, as mentioned. If the desire
to defecate is resisted, then this leads to activation of
the pudendal nerve, which sends signals to the external
anal sphincter, increasing its tone. There is also activation of ascending pathways to the sensory cortex,
enabling the subject to distinguish between solid and

▼

C

gaseous material in the rectum. If there is solid, descending pathways reinforce the external sphincter. If the content is gas, the descending pathways lead to relaxation of the sphincter and expulsion of the gas.

8. When does involuntary defecation occur?

This occurs when the rectal pressure is greater than 55 mmHg. This may occur either because of a voluminous content, or in the presence of colonic spasm and diarrhoea.

The reflex defecation triggered by this pressure rise also occurs in the spinal patient.

9. Summarise the involvement of ANS in the maintenance of continence and defecation.

- PNS: relaxes the internal sphincter
- SNS: stimulates tonic contraction of the internal sphincter

10. Which physiologic mechanisms are involved in the maintenance of faecal continence?

- Sympathetically-mediated tonic contraction of the internal anal sphincter
- The pudendal nerve also maintains tonic contraction of the external sphincter
- Thus, contraction of the sphincters maintains an anal pressure of 40–90 mmHg
- The pubo-rectalis sling of the pelvic floor maintains an anorectal angle of 120°
- Resting intra-abdominal pressure provides a lateral force on the slit-like anal canal, closing it off

COLON

C

CONTROL OF VENTILATION

1. What are the main functions of the lung?

- *Oxygenation*
- *Ventilation:* elimination of carbon dioxide
- *Acid-base balance:* forms the respiratory component to acid-base homeostasis
- *Endocrine:* production of angiotensin converting enzyme

2. Broadly speaking, which parts of the brain are responsible for controlling the rate and depth of ventilation?

- *The brainstem:* pons and medulla involved mainly. These give ventilation its *automacity* and *rhythmical* nature
- *Cerebral cortex:* this gives some voluntary control

3. Which parts of the brainstem have been identified as being particularly important? Outline the role that each plays in control.

Note that these areas of the brainstem have collectively been termed the *respiratory centre.* They consist of:

- *Medullary respiratory centre:* found in the reticular formation. Composed of a *dorsal* group (involved in inspiration) and a *ventral* group (involved in expiration). The expiratory area in the ventral group is not normally active during quiet respiration, since expiration is predominantly a passive process
- *Apneustic area:* located in the pons. This area is thought to prolong the inspiratory phase of the respiratory cycle
- *Pneumotaxic area:* also located in the pons. This inhibits the activity of the inspiratory area of the medulla. It may be involved in 'fine tuning' of respiratory rate, depth and rhythm

▼

4. Which physiologic variables form the basis for control of ventilation? Place them in order of importance.

- *PaCO$_2$:* the most important regulatory factor
- *PaO$_2$*
- *pH of the blood and CSF:* has some influence above and beyond the PaCO$_2$

5. How are changes in these parameters detected?

Through central and peripheral chemoreceptors that stimulate the activity of the brainstem respiratory centre.

6. Where are these receptors located?

- *Central chemoreceptors:* located at the ventral surface of the medulla. These are sensitive to changes in *PaCO$_2$*
- *Peripheral chemoreceptors:* found in the carotid and aortic bodies. These are sensitive mainly to a fall of *PaO$_2$ and pH*, and sensitive to a rise in *PaCO$_2$*.

7. By what mechanism are central chemoceptors sensitive to changes in the PaCO$_2$?

These chemoreceptors are influenced indirectly. Arterial CO$_2$ diffuses into the CSF and dissolves. This produces protons (H$^+$), which then stimulate the central chemoceptor. Therefore, the increased ventilation blows off CO$_2$.

8. Do you know of any other factors influencing the pattern of ventilation?

Yes! The pattern of ventilation is also influenced by the signals from a number of receptors located in and around the respiratory apparatus.

- *Mechanical receptors:* such as pulmonary stretch receptors and *J* receptors. The former are involved in the *Hering-Breuer inflation reflex*, where distension of the lung leads to slowing of inspiration and increased expiratory time. The J receptors are located in the airways close to capillaries, and are thought to stimulate inspiration following and increase in pulmonary blood flow

- *Others:* such irritant receptors in the lungs and nasopharynx, as well as chest wall receptors

9. Below is a graph of the variation in the minute ventilation with the PaO_2. What do the lines A, B and C represent?

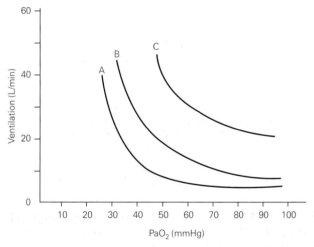

From Berne RM, Levy MN. Principles of Physiology, 3rd edition, 2000, London, with permission from Elsevier

The three lines represent the ventilatory response to changes in the PaO_2 at different $PaCO_2$s. From line A to C there is a progressive increase in the $PaCO_2$.

10. Draw a similar graph of how the ventilatory response varies with the $PaCO_2$ at *different* PaO_2s.

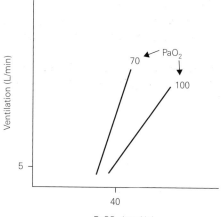

Effect of O_2 and CO_2 ventilatory response. The normal ventilatory response to CO_2 is enhanced by hypoxia; both the threshold (extrapolated X-intercept) and the sensitivity (slope of response) are affected.

From Berne RM, Levy MN. Principles of Physiology, 3rd edition, 2000, London, with permission from Elsevier

11. What happens to the PaO_2, $PaCO_2$ and arterial pH during exercise?

- *PaO_2:* there is usually a slight increase, but during strenuous and persistent exercise, it may fall slightly
- *$PaCO_2$:* this changes little and in strenuous exercise may fall
- *pH:* this remains constant. Even during heavy exercise, buffer systems ensure that lactic acidosis has minimal impact on the overall pH of the blood

Therefore, during moderate exercise, there is surprisingly little variation in all of the above parameters, despite vast increases in the minute ventilation.

C

12. If these physiologic parameters are so consistent during exercise, then what is the stimulus for a rise in the minute ventilation during exercise?

This is not known, but a number of suggestions have been put forward, such as increased limb movement, or oscillations in the partial pressures of the respiratory gases.

CORONARY CIRCULATION

C

1. Where do the coronary arteries originate?

Both the right and left coronary arteries arise directly from the ascending aorta at the aortic sinuses located just above the leaflets of the aortic valve (also known as the sinuses of Valsalva).

2. What is the rate of coronary flow at rest?

70–80 ml/min per 100 g of cardiac tissue. During exercise, this can increase to 300–400 ml/min per 100 g.

3. What percentage of the CO does the heart receive?

4–5%.

4. Given that there is a high myocardial oxygen demand at rest, what functional adaptations ensure that supply meets demand?

Note that the myocardial oxygen consumption is in the order of 8 ml per 100 g of tissue. This is around 20 times that of skeletal muscle. Functional adaptations to ensure adequate oxygen delivery include:

- *High capillary density:* producing a very high surface area for oxygen delivery, and there is high blood flow per unit weight of myocardium
- *High oxygen extraction ratio:* the myocardium extracts around 70% of the oxygen that is delivered to it from the coronary flow. In contrast, the body average is only 25%
- *Efficient metabolic hyperaemia:* myocardial metabolites generated during situations of increased exercise and oxygen demand have a strong influence on control of blood flow
- During exercise, the increased oxygen demand is met predominantly through an increase in the rate of flow rather than an increase in the oxygen extraction ratio

C

5. Look at the graph below, showing the pattern of coronary flow during different phases of the cardiac cycle. What is your interpretation of what is happening? What causes this phenomenon?

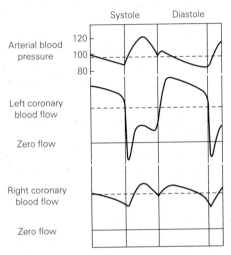

From Smith JJ, Kampire JP. Circulatory Physiology–the Essentials, 3rd edition, Lippincott, Williams & Wilkins

- This shows that coronary flow is greatest during diastole (accounting for 80% of the flow), unlike other vascular beds. The lowest flow is during isovolumetric contraction
- This occurs due to mechanical compression of the coronary vessels during systole, such that there is reversal of the transmural pressure gradient across the wall of the vessel, leading to momentary occlusion

6. What factors are important in the control of coronary blood flow (CBF)?

There are two main influential factors:

- *Metabolic factors:* the dominant controlling process. Some of the products of myocardial metabolism, such as CO_2, prostaglandins and adenosine produce coronary vasodilatation
- *Neural control:* β_2-adrenoceptor stimulation by vasomotor sympathetic nerves leads to coronary vasodilatation. Any neurally-induced coronary vasodilatation is overcome by metabolic factors

7. How does the coronary flow alter with changes of perfusion pressure?

Between perfusion pressures of 60–180 mmHg, the coronary flow is relatively constant. This is known as *autoregulation.*

8. How does this come about?

There are a number of theories. Theses include:

- *Myogenic theory:* increased transmural pressure caused by a rise in the perfusion pressure stretches arteriole myocytes. This stimulates their reflex contraction, producing vasoconstriction. This phenomenon maintains a steady flow despite the rising pressure
- *Vasdilator washout:* transient arteriolar dilatation following a rise in the perfusion pressure also washes out some vasdilators, such as adenosine. Therefore, they can no longer promote further dilatation in the face of rising pressures

9. Why does a sudden occlusion of CBF lead to MI?

Coronary vessels can be considered to be end vessels with little anastomoses between them. At the arteriolar level, branches of the coronaries do communicate, but

C

not enough to sustain the blood supply during acute occlusion. Chronic obstruction, however, leads to the progressive development of collateral vessels that relieve some of the occlusive effects.

FETAL CIRCULATION

F

1. Describe the stages in the passage of blood through the fetal circulation.

- Oxygenated blood enters the fetus from the placenta through the umbilical vein

- About 50% of the blood in the umbilical vein passes into the liver, and goes through the hepatic sinusoids. This eventually enters the inferior vena cava (IVC)

- The other 50% of the umbilical venous blood bypasses the liver via the *ductus venosus* to enter the IVC directly

- From the IVC, the blood enters the right atrium

- It is directed by the septum secundum through the *foramen ovale* and *into the left atrium*. It undergoes mixing with the small amount of deoxygenated blood returning from the lungs through the pulmonary veins

- From the left atrium, blood is ejected into the left ventricle, and eventually into the systemic circulation through the aorta

- A small amount of right atrial blood does not pass through the foramen ovale, but is ejected into the right ventricle, and into the pulmonary trunk

- The vast majority of this pulmonary arterial blood enters the aorta through the *ductus arteriosus*. The rest enters the lungs

- Of the blood that eventually enters the descending aorta, about half supplies the lower body, and the other half enters the umbilical arteries for return back to the placenta

- The diagram below summarises these events:

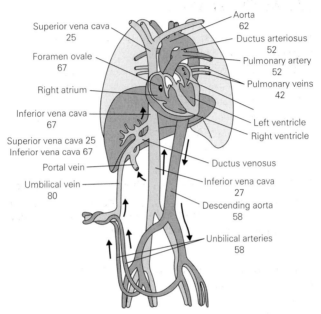

Superior vena cava
25

Foramen ovale
67

Right atrium

Inferior vena cava
67

Superior vena cava 25
Inferior vena cava 67

Portal vein

Umbilical vein
80

Aorta
62

Ductus arteriosus
52

Pulmonary artery
52

Pulmonary veins
42

Left ventricle

Right ventricle

Ductus venosus

Inferior vena cava
27

Descending aorta
58

Unbilical arteries
58

The number refers to oxygen saturation of the blood in %.

From Berne RM, Levy MN. Principles of Physiology, 3rd edition, 2000, London, with permission from Elsevier

2. What changes occur to the fetal circulation following birth?

- *Closure of the three main shunts:* foramen ovale, ductus venosus and ductus arteriosus
- *Closure and degeneration of the umbilical vessels*
- *Fall in pulmonary vascular resistance (PVR):* following aeration of the lungs. This leads to a rise in the pulmonary blood flow. In the first few postnatal months, there is a progressive fall in the PVR
- *Reversal of ventricular wall thickness:* the reduction in the PVR to sub-systemic levels leads to thinning of right ventricular wall compared to the left

GLOMERULAR FILTRATION AND RENAL CLEARANCE

G

1. What factors determine whether a molecule is filtered at the glomerulus?

- *Molecular size:* small molecules such as urea and glucose are filtered freely. The cut off size is about 40 Å

- *Molecular charge:* due to the negative charge of the glomerular basement membrane, negatively charged molecules, like proteins, are not filtered

2. What is meant by the *renal clearance* of a substance?

The renal clearance represents the volume of the plasma from which all of a substance has been removed and excreted in the urine, per unit time.

3. How can the renal clearance be calculated?

From the equation:

$$C = \frac{U \cdot V}{P}$$

where

C = clearance of substance in mlmin^{-1}
U = urinary concentration of the substance
V = urine flow rate per minute
P = plasma concentration of the substance

4. From which physical law is this equation derived?

The concept of renal clearance is based on the law of *mass balance*. With respect to the kidney, this states that:

Amount of substance X excreted =
  Amount filtered − Amount reabsorbed
  + Amount secreted

▼

G

5. Under what circumstances does the renal clearance of a substance equal the glomerular filtration rate (GFR)?

The clearance of a substance is the same as the GFR when that substance is excreted purely by the process of filtration.

In that situation, the amount filtered = amount excreted

$$GFR \cdot P = U \cdot V$$
$$\text{Thus, } GFR = \frac{U \cdot V}{P}$$

6. Do you know of a substance that is excreted purely through glomerular filtration, enabling it to be used for measurements of the GFR?

Yes, the polyfructose molecule inulin. It is used for measurement of the GFR because the volume of plasma completely cleared of inulin per unit time is equal to the volume of plasma filtered per unit time.

7. What physiologic properties make a substance suitable for measurements of the GFR?

- It must be filtered freely at the glomerulus
- It must not undergo secretion or reabsorption by the tubules
- It must not be metabolised by the kidney
- It must not inherently alter the GFR

8. What is the practical disadvantage to using inulin for GFR measurements?

It must undergo continuous intravenous infusion.

9. What is the most common way of measuring the GFR?

By measuring 24-hour urinary creatinine excretion. This molecule is endogenously produced at a generally constant rate. It is not perfect for GFR measurements since it is secreted by the tubules to a slight degree.

10. What is the difference between *creatine* and *creatinine*?

- *Creatine:* this is an amino acid stored in muscle and brain tissue. It acts as a ready and rapid source of phosphate groups when muscle exercises. During periods of minimal activity, it is phosphorylated into creatine phosphate. This phosphate is released during activity
- *Creatinine:* this is the anhydride of creatine and is formed as a waste product of creatine metabolism

11. What is the normal range of creatinine clearance?

The normal range is 80–110 mlmin^{-1} and declines with increasing age.

12. What normally happens to glucose following filtration at the glomerulus?

The filtered load of glucose normally undergoes complete reabsorption by cells of the proximal tubule. Therefore none is found in the urine.

G

13. Below is a graph of glucose transport in the nephron versus plasma glucose concentration. What does it show?

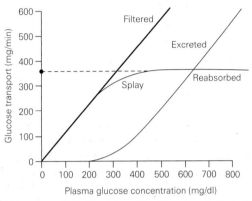

Adapted from NMS: Physiology, 4th edition, Bullock, Boyle & Wang, 2001, Lippincott, Williams & Wilkins

This shows that below a filtered load of glucose of about $400 \, \text{mg} \, \text{min}^{-1}$, all of the glucose filtered is absorbed by the proximal tubule (through an active process). Above this filtration load, glucose starts to appear in the urine since the ability of the tubular cells to reabsorb glucose is overcome. This maximum absorptive rate is called the *tubular transport maximum* (T_m). The *splay* on the graph is due to the variations in the glucose handling of individual nephrons.

IMMOBILIZATION

1. Which systems of the body show physiologic changes following prolonged immobilization?

- The musculoskeletal system
- Cardiovascular system
- Autonomic nervous system
- The extra-cellular fluid compartment
- There are also changes in overall body composition of fat and protein

2. What are these changes in the overall body composition that you have mentioned?

- *Reduction in the lean body mass:* this is seen as an increase in the excretion of nitrogen after the 5th day of bed rest. The level of protein catabolism falls after several weeks, but is still higher than normal
- *Increase of adipose tissue deposition:* as a replacement for loss of muscle mass
- *Increased potassium excretion:* since this is the major intracellular cation and especially rich in muscle, loss of potassium is an indicator of loss of total body lean tissue mass

3. How long after continued bed rest are cardiovascular changes seen?

About three weeks.

4. What are these changes?

- *Increase in heart rate:* after three weeks, the rate increases about half a beat per minute per day of immobilization
- *Reduction of stroke volume:* this is associated with a measure of cardiac atrophy
- *CO and arterial pressure are maintained:* owing to the conflicting changes above

- *Adaptations to postural changes are impaired:* this is because of impairment of the inotropic and CO response to a fall in the arterial pressure, despite an exaggerated peripheral vascular response. There is also a reduction in the overall activity of the ANS, leading to a blunting of cardiovascular responses

5. What happens to the musculoskeletal system following three weeks of bed rest?

- *Demineralisation of bone:* observed as an increase in the urinary excretion of calcium, phosphate and hydroxyprolene. There is a disproportionate degree of demineralisation of load-bearing bones, such as the calcaneum. The endocrine changes that account for this are not fully understood, but they can be reversed by rhythmical limb movements, even when supine
- *Muscular changes:* there is a reduction of muscle bulk and muscle power, especially from the lower limbs

6. What happens to the blood volume during prolonged immobilization?

After three weeks, there may be a fall of up to 600 ml. This is due to loss of plasma volume, with minimal fall in the circulating red cell volume. Also contributes to reduced cardiovascular responses to postural changes.

7. Apart from the long-term changes mentioned above, what are the other major risks of prolonged bed rest?

- *Increased risk of DVT:* this forms one of the tenets of Virchow's triad
- *Increased risk of decubitus ulcers:* especially over superficially bony areas, such as the sacrum. Risk increases if the individual is incapacitated and cannot change position in bed

LIVER

L

1. What are the functions of the liver?

Functions may be divided into: storage functions, metabolic, endocrine, coagulation, and other

- *Storage:* vitamins D, A, K, folate and B_{12} and Iron (as ferratin)
- *Metabolic:*
  - *Carbohydrate:* glycogen storage, gluconeogenesis
  - *Lipid:* formation of ketone bodies, cholesterol, phospholipid and lipoprotein synthesis, conversion of protein and carbohydrate into lipid
  - *Protein:* protein synthesis (especially plasma proteins, like albumin and complement), deamination of amino acids and formation of urea
- *Endocrine:* involved in breakdown of the steroid hormones
- *Coagulation:* synthesis of clotting factors, prothrombin, fibrinogen and antithrombin III
- *Other functions:* generation of heat, breakdown of red cells and is central to the reticuloendothelial system (RES), drug metabolism and site of extramedullary haemopoesis in adults

2. What percentage of the CO reaches the liver?

About 30%.

3. By which route does most of this blood reach the liver?

Via the portal vein from the gut. This accounts for 70% of hepatic blood flow.

4. List some important basic liver function tests.

- *Bilirubin:* both free and conjugated

LIVER

- *Liver enzymes:* aspartate aminotransferase (AST) and alanine aminotransferase (ALT) these are released by injured hepatocytes
  - Alkaline phosphatase: raised in cholestasis
  - γ-glutamyl transferase: non specific marker
- *Plasma proteins:* albumin: reduced in chronic liver disease
  - Globulins: as above
- *Clotting studies:* leads to abnormal prothrombin time (PT) and activated partial thromboplastin time (APTT)

5. Which tumour marker is associated with hepatocellular carcinoma?

α-fetoprotein.

6. How much bile does the liver secrete daily?

About 500 ml per day.

7. What is its basic composition?

- *97% water*
- *0.7% bile salts:* sodium and potassium salts of bile acids
- *0.2% bile pigments:* bilirubin and biliverdin. They give bile its characteristic colour
- *2% other:* fatty acids, cholesterol and lecithin

8. What are the four major bile salts?

- Cholic acid
- Chenodeoxycholic acid
- Deoxycholic acid
- Lithocholic acid

The latter two molecules are derived from bacterial action on the former two in the colon.

Note that these agents are derived from cholesterol, and as with steroid hormones, share the same cyclopentanoperhydrophenantherene ring nucleus that characterises this family of molecules.

9. What is the major function of the bile salts?

They are responsible for the emulsification of fat in the chyme by the formation of micelles. This aids in their absorption. It follows that they are also important for the absorption of the fat-soluble vitamins A, D, E, and K. Most of the bile acids undergo entero-hepatic circulation.

10. Where does bilirubin come from?

The main source is from the breakdown of the haem component of haemoglobin in the RES. A little is formed in the liver itself following the metabolism of various haemoproteins such as cytochrome P-450.

11. How does it reach the liver and what happens to it when it does?

The circulating, insoluble bilirubin reaches the liver bound to albumin. Here it undergoes conjugation to bilirubin diglucuronide with the aid of the enzyme glucuronyl transferase.

Most of this conjugated bilirubin enters the bile and into the gut. A small amount enters the circulation, where it reaches the urine.

The bilirubin in the terminal ileum is converted into urobilinogen, which is excreted in the faeces (as sterocobilin). Some of this also enters the urine (~10% of the total).

12. How high does the serum bilirubin have to get before jaundice appears?

Above $35\,mmolL^{-1}$.

13. What is the broad classification for the causes of jaundice? `

- *Excess production of bilirubin:* e.g. haemolytic anaemia
- *Decreased uptake into hepatocytes:* Gilbert's syndrome
- *Abnormal conjugation:* prematurity, Crigler-Najjar
- *Cholestasis:* due to obstruction to the excretion of conjugated bile – produces a conjugated hyperbilirubinaemia. Obstruction may be intra- or extra-hepatic

14. What does the bilirubin level tell you about the aetiology?

In cases of cholestasis, the serum bilirubin may be up to $500 \, \text{mmolL}^{-1}$. The lowest levels are generally seen in cases of 'pre-hepatic' jaundice, such as intra-vascular haemolysis.

15. How is gall bladder contraction regulated?

In response to fatty food entering the duodenum, cholecystokinin (CCK) is released from the duodenal mucosa. This stimulates gall bladder contraction and relaxation of the sphincter of Oddi. Bile secretion is also stimulated by CCK, gastrin and secretin.

MECHANICS OF BREATHING I – VENTILATION

1. What is the FiO$_2$ of atmospheric air?

0.21, since 21% of the atmosphere is made up of oxygen.

2. What is the difference between minute ventilation and alveolar ventilation?

- Minute ventilation is the total volume of air entering the respiratory tree every minute, and is equal to *Tidal Volume (TV) × Respiratory Rate*
- Alveolar ventilation is the volume of gas entering the alveoli each minute. It takes into account the *anatomic dead space.* This volume of inspired air does not come into contact with respiratory epithelium. Alveolar ventilation is equal to *(TV − Anatomic dead space) × Respiratory rate.* In a resting 70 kg adult it is about $(0.5 - 0.15) \times 12 = 4.2 \, \mathrm{L \, min^{-1}}$

Thus, the alveolar ventilation is a more accurate measure of the level of ventilation since it takes into account only the volume of gas that interfaces with the respiratory epithelium. It can be seen that if a subject takes rapid, shallow breaths, they will become hypoxaemic despite numerically adequate minute ventilation.

3. What is meant by the *oxygen cascade*?

This term describes the incremental drops in the pO$_2$ from the atmosphere to the arterial blood.

4. What are the changes in the oxygen cascade?

- *Atmospheric air:* PO$_2$ = 21 kPa
- *Tracheal air:* PO$_2$ = 19.8 kPa
- *Alveolar gas:* PO$_2$ = 14.0 kPa
- *Arterial blood gas:* PO$_2$ = 13.3 kPa

5. What about the changes in the partial pressure of CO_2 along the respiratory tree?

- *Atmospheric air:* $PCO_2 = 0.03\,kPa$
- *Alveolar air:* $PCO_2 = 5.3\,kPa$
- *Arterial gas:* $PCO_2 = 5.3\,kPa$
- *Venous gas:* $PCO_2 = 6.1\,kPa$
- *Exhaled air:* $PCO_2 = 4\,kPa$

6. Why is there virtually no alveolar-arterial PCO_2 difference, unlike oxygen?

Carbon dioxide has a very high water solubility compared to oxygen, with rapid and efficient diffusion across the respiratory epithelium.

7. Under what conditions does this difference increase?

Under the pathological conditions of a Ventilation/Perfusion mismatch, and when there is an increase in CO_2 production.

8. Which equation defines the relationship between the PaO_2 and the $PaCO_2$?

The relationship is given by the *alveolar gas equation*. In its simplified form this states that

$$PaO_2 = P_iO_2 - PaCO_2/R$$

where PiO_2 = Inspired PO_2; R = Respiratory exchange ratio, normally 0.8

This shows how the partial pressures of the two respiratory gases influence each other inversely.

MECHANICS OF BREATHING II – RESPIRATORY CYCLE

M

1. List the muscles of inspiration, starting with the most important.

- *Diaphragm*
- *External intercostals*
- *Accessory muscles:* sternocleidomastoid, scalene group, strap muscles of the neck

2. What is the nerve supply of the diaphragm, and what is its root value?

The supply is from the phrenic nerves, from C_3, C_4, and C_5.

3. What part do the external intercostals play during inspiration?

When they contract, the ribs are pulled *upwards and forwards.* Rib elevation leads to a 'bucket handle' motion that increases the lateral dimension of the thorax. A forward pull to the ribs increases the antero-posterior diameter of the thorax.

4. During quiet respiration, which are the chief muscles of expiration?

There are none; due to the elastic properties of the lung and chest wall, expiration is a *passive process.* Note that the volume of air left in the lung during a quiet expiration is the *functional residual capacity (FRC).*

5. What about the expiratory muscles during exercise or a forceful expiration?

The most important expiratory muscles in these situations are the abdominal muscles *(rectus abdominis, internal/external obliques, and transversus abdominis).*

The internal intercostals aid in this process.

▼

M

6. Draw a graph showing the changes in the intrapleural and alveolar pressures during the respiratory cycle. Explain the changes seen.

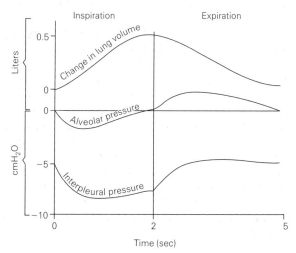

From NMS: Physiology, 4th edition, Bullock, Boyle & Wang, 2001, Lippincott, Williams & Wilkins

- During a normal inspiration, the lung volume reaches the TV
- At the end of expiration, just before another breath in, the alveolar pressure is at atmospheric pressure. At this stage, since there is no pressure difference between the alveolus and the atmosphere, there is no airflow into the lung
- Increasing the volume of the thoracic cavity during inspiration causes the alveolar pressure to drop below atmospheric pressure (by about 1 cmH$_2$O). This pressure difference causes air to flow into the lung, increasing the lung volume
- During expiration, the natural elastic recoil of the lung compresses the alveoli, with resulting increase

▼

in the alveolar pressure to above atmospheric. This leads to airflow out of the lungs

- The point just before inspiration marks the *equilibrium point*. The tendency of the lung to collapse due to its elastic recoil is prevented by the forces that hold the chest wall in position. The constant elastic recoil of the lung leads to a resting intrapleural pressure of $5\,cmH_2O$ below atmospheric (or $-5\,cmH_2O$)

- Note that the lung is held in position next to the chest wall by the thin film of the intrapleural fluid

- During inspiration, the intrapleural pressure falls further for two reasons: firstly, as the lung expands, the elastic recoil increases. This increases the pull on the chest wall, dropping the intrapleural pressure further. Secondly, the fall in the alveolar pressure is transmitted to the intrapleural space, increasing the pressure drop

- During expiration, the intrapleural pressure returns to its resting level

7. Under what circumstance does the intrapleural pressure become positive?

This occurs during forced expiration.

M

MECHANICS OF BREATHING III – COMPLIANCE AND ELASTANCE

1. What is meant by lung compliance?

This is defined as the change in lung volume per unit change in pressure. Thus, it is a measure of the ease with which the lung *inflates*.

2. What is the overall compliance of the lung?

$200 \, \text{ml/cmH}_2\text{O}$.

3. Below is the pressure-volume relationship of an isolated lung block. How is the compliance calculated from this plot?

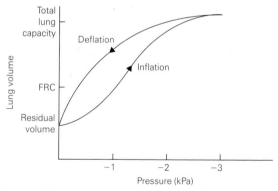

From Yentis S, Hirsch N, Smith GB. Anaesthesia & Intensive Care:
A to Z, 2nd edition, 2000, Butterworth Heinemann

The compliance is calculated from the slope of the straight line joining any two points on the curve.

4. Looking at the graph, how does the compliance differ during inspiration and expiration?

During expiration, the compliance of the lung is *greater*. It can be seen that the volume is greater for a given pressure.

5. What is this phenomenon called?

Hysteresis.

6. Below is an imaginary system of two balloons connected by a tube. One balloon is much larger than the other. What happens to the volumes of the balloons when tap A is closed and tap B is opened to allow mixing of gases between the two?

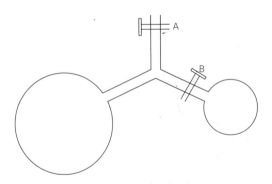

The smaller balloon deflates, and the air contained enters the larger one.

7. What is the explanation for what happens?

The explanation lies with Laplace's Law. This states that the transmural pressure,

$$P = \frac{2T}{r}$$

where T = wall tension; r = radius.

The smaller the radius of the sphere, the greater the
transmural pressure (or trans-pulmonary pressure in
the case of the lung) required to oppose the wall tension to prevent collapse.

8. How is this example related to an understanding of lung compliance?

The smaller the alveolus, the greater the inflation
pressure required to overcome the surface (or wall)
tension during inflation. Thus, the best way to reduce
the inflation pressure required to expand an alveolus is
to reduce the surface tension. In other words, the best
way to increase the compliance of an alveolus, and make
its inflation easier, is to reduce the surface tension.

9. How is the compliance reduced *in vivo*?

Through the secretion of *pulmonary surfactant*. This
reduces the surface tension of the fluid lining the alveolus, and in doing so reduces the compliance of the
lung, as seen by the Law of Laplace.

10. What is this secretion composed of?

It is composed of a mixture of lipid and proteins. The
most important lipid constituents are *dipalmitylphos-
phatidylcholine* and *cholesterol*.

11. What is its source?

It is produced by the lung's Type II pneumocytes.

12. Summarise the functions of pulmonary surfactant.

- By lowering the surface tension of the alveoli, it
  increases the compliance of the lung, and reduces
  the work of breathing

▼

- Stabilises smaller alveoli, preventing their collapse during deflation. This has the overall effect of preventing atelectasis
- Keeps alveoli dry, by reducing transudation of fluid from the interstitium

13. Which diseases can alter lung compliance?

- *Increased compliance:* chronic obstructive pulmonary disease (COPD), old age (note, this is not a disease!)
- *Decreased compliance:* pulmonary fibrosis and restrictive lung disease, pulmonary venous congestion, pulmonary oedema (including adult respiratory distress syndrome (ARDS))

14. How does it vary under normal physiological situations?

- *Variations in the respiratory cycle:* compliance is greater during expiration
- *Position:* lung compliance is less lying down due to less FRC

15. What is elastance?

This is 1/compliance. Thus, it is a measure of the elastic recoil of the lung.

16. What generates this force?

- The elastic properties of the elastin and collagen network of the lung
- Surface tension at the alveolus

MECHANICS OF BREATHING IV – AIRWAY RESISTANCE

1. Which law defines the resistance to flow through any tube?

Poiseuille's law, which states that:

$$R = \frac{8\eta L}{\pi r^4}$$

where R = resistance; η = viscosity of air or fluid in the tube; L = length of tube; r = radius of tube

2. What is the relationship of the airway resistance to the magnitude of airflow?

This is defined by the equation:

$$V = \frac{\Delta P}{R}$$

where ΔP = driving pressure.

The driving pressure for airflow to occur is normally very low, typically 1–2 cmH$_2$O.

3. Where are the sites of greatest airways resistance?

- *Upper airways:* nose, mouth, pharynx and larynx. Accounts for about 50% of airway resistance
- Trachea, and bronchi down to the seventh generation (medium sized bronchi)
- Note that at the individual level, the smaller airways have the highest resistance, but since there are so many of these in the lungs, their overall cross-sectional area is very large

4. What physiologic factors influence the diameter of the airways, and hence airways resistance?

- *Lung volumes*
- *Respiratory secretions*
- *Activity of airway smooth muscle cells:* determined by the ANS and chemical mediators

5. In what way does the volume of the lung determine the resistance of the airway?

The greater the lung volume, the less the overall airway resistance. This is due to the effects of *radial traction*. The larger the lung volume, the greater the elastic recoil forces across the airways. The elastic recoil of an airway pulls the others around it open, increasing their calibre and reducing their resistance by the Poiseuille equation. At lower lung volumes, the effect of this radial traction is diminished, reducing the calibre of the airways. Note that only airways that are unsupported by mural cartilage are subject to the effects of radial traction.

Radial traction is due to the elastin and collagen in the airways, and is lost in emphysema. This leads to air trapping and increased lung volumes.

6. What happens to the airways at very low lung volumes, near the FRC?

Below the FRC, the smaller airways collapse due to the effects mentioned above. The volume at which this normal collapse occurs is called the *closing volume*. In young subjects, it occurs between the FRC and the residual volume (RV), and explains why not all the gas in the lung can be exhaled. The closing volume increases with age, and in the elderly, it may be above the FRC.

M

M

7. Below is a maximal flow-volume loop taken from a normal individual during forced expiration and inspiration. What is represented at point A? What does the downward slope B represents?

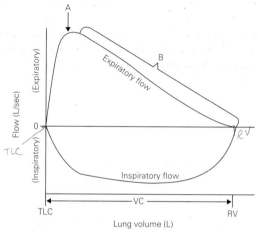

From NMS: Physiology, 4th edition, Bullock, Boyle & Wang, 2001, Lippincott, Williams & Wilkins

- Point A is the peak flow rate
- Slope B is the forced expiratory volume (FEV). The FEV in 1 s can be measured from this line

8. What is meant by *dynamic airway compression*, and how does it relate to slope B above?

Dynamic airway compression is collapse of unsupported airways that occurs during forced expiration. During this manoeuvre, intrapleural pressures may reach $+30\,cmH_2O$. This is much greater than the pressure in some parts of the airways. Consequently this high pressure compresses these airways, preventing further airflow out of them.

▼

The slope B during expiration is 'effort independent' in any one individual, and reaches a ceiling irrespective of the expiratory force generated. This is due to the effects of dynamic airways compression limiting the rate of expiration. The greater the expiratory force generated, the greater the airway compression limiting flow.

9. Draw a graph showing how the flow-volume loop alters in COPD and restrictive lung disease compared to normality. What happens to the FEV and FEV_1 under these circumstances?

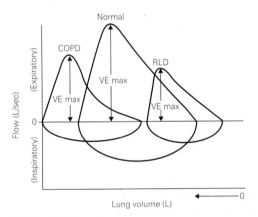

RLD=Restrictive lung disease

From NMS: Physiology, 4th edition, Bullock, Boyle & Wang, 2001, Lippincott, Williams & Wilkins

- Note that in COPD, the total lung capacity (TLC), FRC and RV are greater due to gas trapping following loss of radial traction. Peak flow is reduced due to airways obstruction and reduced lung elastance. FEV_1/FVC is reduced
- In restrictive lung disease, all the lung volumes are reduced, but the FEV_1/FVC is normal or increased

MICROCIRCULATION I

1. What is this equation, and in simple terms, what is it describing?

$$J_v = L_pS\{(P_c - P_i) - \sigma(\pi_p - \pi_i)\}$$

This is the *Starling equation* and describes the factors that determine the flow of water across capillary walls.

2. So, basically, what is it saying?

It states that the net filtration of water across a capillary wall is proportional to the difference between the hydraulic and osmotic forces across the vessel wall where:

- P_c: capillary filtration pressure
- P_i: interstitial pressure
- π_p: colloid oncotic (osmotic) pressure
- π_i: interstitial oncotic pressure

3. What are the other symbols in the equation, and what do they mean?

- L_p: hydraulic conductance. This is the filtration rate per unit change of pressure across the membrane
- S: surface area of the vessel wall
- σ: the reflection coefficient. This is simply a measure of how leaky the membrane is. This measures about 0.8, meaning that only 80% of the potential oncotic pressure is exerted across the vessel wall

4. Can you name some factors that determine the P_c across a capillary wall?

- *Distance along the capillary:* going from the arterial to the venous side of the capillary, there is a fall in the pressure. Typically, at the arterial end it is 35 mmHg, and at the venous end, 20 mmHg
- The resistances of the arterioles and venules at either end of the capillary

▼

- *Gravity:* both arterial and venous pressures increase below the heart

5. Can you elaborate on how the resistances of surrounding arterioles and venules affect the P_c of the capillary?

In basic terms the greater the resistance of the surrounding vessel, the lower the P_c. What is important though, is the ratio of the resistance of the arteriole to the venule (R_a/R_v).

- The greater the R_a/R_v the lower the P_c. When the arteriole is constricted, the P_c is closer to the (lower) pressure in the venule
- The lower the R_a/R_v the higher the P_c, because the arteriole is less constricted, its pressure has a greater influence on the P_c

And so it follows that, from the Starling equation, the greater the P_c, the greater rate of filtration of water across the vessel wall into the interstitium.

6. Can you name another filtration process that is influenced heavily by the resistance ratios?

The net filtration of water across the glomerulus is also influenced by the pre-to-post capillary resistance ratios. This leads to alterations in not only the GFR, but also the filtration fraction (the proportion of water passing through the glomerulus that is filtered through). Although other Starling forces are important in determining filtration across the glomerulus, the main point of control of the GFR is through alterations in the vascular resistances.

7. Give a normal value for the colloid osmotic pressure.

25 mmHg.

8. Which proteins are most important in exerting the plasma colloid osmotic pressure?

- *Albumin:* with a molecular weight of 69,000
- *γ-globulins:* with a combined molecular weight of 150,000

9. What about the interstitium?

The major proteins in the interstitium are:

- Collagen
- Proteoglycans
- Hyaluronate

These have a positive influence on both the osmotic pressure and the interstitial fluid pressure. (As the interstitial proteins take up water, they swell, increasing the interstitial pressure.)

MICROCIRCULATION II

M

1. What is oedema (edema)?

This is defined as the abnormal accumulation of fluid in the *extravascular* space.

2. What are two broad types, and how may they be distinguished?

- *Transudate:* due to imbalances in the hydrostatic forces of the Starling equation
- *Exudate:* occurs following an increase in the capillary permeability

The main difference (that can be used to aid diagnosis of the aetiology) is that an exudates is rich in protein and fibrinogen.

3. What are the main causes?

The main causes are categorised according to the variables in the Starling equation:

- *Reduced colloid osmotic pressure (π_p):* that occurs with hypoproteinaemic states, such as malnutrition, protein-losing enteropathy and the nephrotic syndrome
- *Increased capillary filtration pressure (P_c):* as in cardiac failure where there is peripheral dependant oedema, ascites and pulmonary oedema. Most commonly, the main culprit is an elevation of the venous pressure, as in deep venous thrombosis. Increased filtration pressure also arises from abnormal retention of salt and water, e.g. renal failure an other causes of hypervolaemia
- *Increased capillary permeability:* leading to the formation of an exudates – which follows an inflammatory process where there is an immune mediated increase in the capillary permeability

- *Lymphatic occlusion:* leading to an accumulation of fluid in the interstitial compartment, e.g. malignant occlusion following lymphatic compression or lymphadenopathy

4. Apart from the increase in the capillary permeability, why else does inflammation promote oedema?

The vasodilatation associated with inflammation increases the capillary filtration pressure (i.e. there is a decrease in the pre-to-post capillary resistance ratio). As seen in *Microcirculation I,* the P_c is closely determined by the pre-to-post capillary resistance ratio.

5. During the inflammatory process, which mediators are responsible for the increase in the capillary permeability?

- *Histamine:* released from mast cells and basophils
- *5-HT:* from platelets
- *Platelet-activating factor:* from neutrophils, basophils and macrophages
- *Others:* $C5_a$, PGE_2, and bradykinin

MICTURITION

M

1. What are the functions of the bladder?

- Collection and low pressure storage of urine
- Expulsion of urine at an appropriate time and place
- Aids in preventing organisms from ascending to the upper urinary tract

2. Outline the innervation of the bladder.

- *PNS:* the bladder's detrusor muscle has a rich parasympathetic supply that causes contraction. These nerves run from spinal segments S2, 3 and 4. It also causes sphincter relaxation
- *SNS:* these travel with the hypogastric nerves from L1, 2 and 3. Leads to α_1 mediated contraction of the sphincter and β_2 mediated relaxation of the detrusor
- These nerves combine to form a plexus at the base of the bladder

3. How is the bladder's sphincteric mechanism arranged in the male?

In males, there are two distinctive systems:

- *Bladder neck mechanism:* this is proximally placed. This not only provides urinary continence, but also prevents retrograde ejaculation
- *Distal sphincter mechanism:* this is a urethra-based system that lies at the apex of the prostate gland. This is able to maintain continence even in the face of injury to the bladder neck mechanism

4. How does this arrangement differ from that of the female?

- *Bladder neck mechanism:* in females, this system is poorly defined and may even be incompetent in the nulliparous

- *Distal sphincter mechanism:* this is relatively more important in females. It is longer than the male counterpart, extending along two-thirds of the urethra

5. At what bladder volume is the first urge to micturate felt?

About 150 ml. At 400 ml, there is a marked sense of fullness.

6. What is the capacity of the bladder?

Around 500 ml.

7. What are the two phases of bladder function?

- Storage phase
- Initiation and controlled voiding

8. What is the important feature of the first phase?

During the storage phase, the bladder shows *receptive relaxation*. This means that the bladder progressively fills and expands without much increase in the intra-vesical pressure.

9. Outline the events during the voiding phase.

- As the bladder fills, afferent activity from stretch receptors increase and passes via the posterior roots of the sacral cord to the brain, thereby mediating the desire to void
- The higher centres are able to intervene at any time during the voiding reflex to stop or re-initiate the process
- During voiding, urethral relaxation precedes detrusor contraction

M

- There is simultaneous relaxation of the pelvic floor muscles
- The neuronal control of this coordinated activity is not fully understood. It is thought that central inhibitory influences acting on sacral centres are removed and voiding is initiated under the influence of pontine medullary centres. This is associated with increased PNS flow to the detrusor muscle, leading to sphincter relaxation and detrusor contraction

10. What happens to the voiding cycle in the spinal patient?

If the spinal cord is transacted above the 5th lumbar segment, the state of *cord bladder* develops. This leads to a state of detrusor-sphincter dyssynergia, where there is simultaneous contraction of the detrusor and urethral sphincter. Voiding still occurs since the sphincter contractions are not prolonged, but there is still a considerable urinary retention.

MICTURITION

MOTOR CONTROL

1. What kinds of coordinated movements does skeletal muscle contraction lead to?

- Voluntary movement
- Reflexes
- Maintenance of posture
- Repetitive and rhythmical movements, e.g. breathing

All of these types of movement are under the control of an *integrated motor system.*

2. What are the components of the motor system that initiate, coordinate and execute these movements?

The components can be thought of as forming an inter-active hierarchy. They consist of:

- *Cerebral cortex:* consisting of the motor cortex and associated areas
- *Subcortical areas:* the cerebellum, basal ganglia and brainstem
- *Spinal cord:* this carries fibres from the cerebral cortex to motoneurones, but is also capable of its own intrinsic reflex activity
- *Motoneurones:* these form the final common pathway
- *Motor units:* the functional contractile unit
- *Receptors and afferent pathways:* these sensory pathways relay information back to the other components, which can in turn adjust movement, e.g. proprioceptive information

3. Where is the motor cortex located?

This is found at the *precentral gyrus* (Brodmann's area 4). This controls contralateral muscular activity. There is also an associated motor cortex, found in Brodmann's areas 6. This helps control movement on both sides of the body.

▼

4. Where in the spinal cord are cell bodies of the motoneurones located?

These are located in the *ventral* horns of the spinal cord. They congregate together as *motor nuclei* in specific parts of this ventral horn depending on whether they supply muscles of the axial or appendicular skeleton, and whether they supply proximal or distal limb muscles.

Note that they may also be found in the brainstem, as the motor nuclei of cranial nerves III, IV, VI and XII.

5. What types of motoneurone are there, and what types of skeletal muscle fibre do they innervate?

- α-*motoneurons:* these are large diameter fibres that innervate the majority of worker fibre. Such fibres are also known as *extrafusal* fibre since they are not encased within connective tissue sheaths. Such α fibres have multiple dendritic processes
- γ-*motoneurons:* these have smaller axons than the above and innervate the *intrafusal* fibres of the muscle spindle

6. Apart from skeletal muscle, what other connections do motoneurones make?

Motoneurones synapse with a number of other type of cell through connections on their cell bodies:

- *Afferent sensory fibres:* such as the afferents from cutaneous receptors that mediate cutaneous reflexes, and muscle spindle afferent fibres that mediate muscle reflexes
- *Descending pathways:* these make synaptic connections directly from higher centres. Such connections may run down in *pyramidal* or *extrapyramidal* pathways
- *Interneurones:* these are the most common kind of synaptic connection onto motoneurones. They are usually found between afferent neurones and

M

motoneurones. They may form *excitatory*, or *inhibitory* connections, and so influence motoneurone activity. One important inhibitory interneurone is the *Renshaw* cell, which is vital for controlling motoneurone firing

7. Define the motor unit.

This consists of a motoneurone and all of the muscle fibres that it innervates. The sizes of the unit vary greatly depending on the type of muscle. Large muscles and those involved in maintaining posture consist of very large units, with many fibres being innervated by one axon. Muscles involved in delicate and precise movements have small units, where only a few fibres are innervated by a single motoneurone.

Note that all of the fibres in any individual unit are of the same type, i.e. fast-twitch, slow-twitch, or fast fatigue-resistant fibres. Thus, whenever a motoneurone fires, *all* of the muscle fibres in that unit contract.

8. What is a reflex?

This is defined as an automatic response to a stimulus.

9. What are the two main types of spinal cord reflex that involve skeletal muscle activity?

- *Withdrawal reflex:* this is mediated by cutaneous nociceptors that connect to afferent pathways that stimulate α-motoneurones. Thus there is automatic contraction of a muscle in response to a painful stimulus. This is a complex polysynaptic pathway that also leads to inhibition of antagonistic muscles to the flexors
- *Stretch reflex:* there is reflex muscle contraction following stretch of the fibres. This is seen most clearly in the *knee jerk* reflex. It is mediated by the action of muscle *spindle* receptors interspersed among the regular muscle fibres

M

10. What types of muscle fibre form muscle spindles?

These are formed from *intrafusal* muscle fibres. Unlike regular muscle fibres, these special fibres that form spindles are located within connective tissue capsules. The ratio of regular fibres to spindle fibres varies according to the function of each muscle.

Note that such spindle fibres lie in *parallel* with the regular, extrafusal fibres.

11. What types of muscle spindle are there?

There are two types, depending on the morphology of the fibre within the spindle capsule:

- *Nuclear bag fibres:* so-called because of the central clustering of their nuclei. They are generally longer and thicker than the nuclear chain fibres
- *Nuclear chain fibres:* the nuclei are arranged as a chain along the fibre

12. How does the afferent innervation arising from each of these differ?

- *Nuclear bag fibres* are connected mainly to Group Ia afferents
- *Nuclear chain fibres* are connected mainly to Group II sensory afferents, which are smaller and slower conducting than the above

13. Describe the steps involved in the muscle stretch (knee jerk) reflex.

- The patellar tendon is stretched following contact with the tendon hammer. This also results in stretch of the quadriceps muscle
- The muscle spindle fibres, which lie in parallel to the regular muscle fibres, are also stretched
- The afferents arising from the spindles discharge, relaying back directly to the α-motoneurone in the ventral horn of the spinal cord

- Thus, there is a *monosynaptic* pathway of connection
- This *excitatory* connection leads to firing of the α-motoneurone, which leads to reflex contraction of the quadriceps
- The spindle afferent fibres also synapse with inhibitory interneurones that inhibit the contraction of the hamstrings

14. What is the role of the γ-motoneurones that innervate muscle spindles?

Stimulation of these fibres causes stretch of the fibres within the spindle without affecting the length of the surrounding extrafusal fibres. Therefore, by altering the initial length of the fibre, there is an alteration in the *sensitivity* of the spindle to the stretching of the rest of the muscle.

MUSCLE I – SKELETAL AND SMOOTH MUSCLE

1. What types of muscle are there in the body?

- *Skeletal:* Striated and voluntary
- *Cardiac:* Striated and involuntary
- *Smooth:* Involuntary

2. What is mechanical summation?

This is when the force of contraction increases through the stimulation of multiple twitch contractions whose individual forces *accumulate.* This only occurs when the muscle is stimulated to contract before it has fully relaxed from a contraction preceding it.

3. What happens to the fibre if there is continuous stimulation?

If the muscle is stimulated at increasing frequency, a twitch contraction becomes a long and continuous *tetanic* contraction. The force generated by tetanus is much greater than that of a twitch. The frequency required to generate a tetanic contraction is called the *tetanic frequency.*

4. What are the basic types of skeletal muscle fibre and mention briefly some of their differences.

- *Type I:* slow twitch fibre that is also slow to fatigue. Contains a high concentration of myoglobin, e.g. soleus muscle
- *Type II:* fast twitch that also fatigues quickly. They have large reserves of glycogen as an energy source, e.g. extraocular muscles. There are two types of fast-twitch fibre depending on their degree of activity

M

5. Draw a sarcomere, and label it.

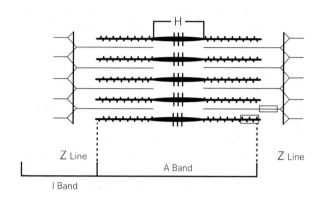

6. What is the function of the T tubule system, and where is it located?

This system is an invagination of the sarcolemma (muscle cell membrane). In skeletal muscle, it is located at the junction of the A and I bands. It also lies adjacent to the sarcoplasmic reticulum (SR), so that there is rapid release of Ca^{2+}.

It is important for the transmission of the action potential across the myofibril.

7. What is the source of intracellular calcium?

Calcium ions are stored in the SR. This is a network of tubules (akin to the endoplasmic reticulum of other cells) that separates the myofibrils. The SR lies against the T tubule network. This point of contact is called the *lateral cistern* of the SR.

Therefore, the action potentials running within the T tubule system can stimulate a rapid release of Ca^{2+} from the SR.

▼

8. List the architectural hierarchy of the skeletal muscle cell.

- The muscle is divided into bundles of fascicles that are separated by a connective tissue sheath
- Each fascicle is composed of bundles of individual muscle fibres separated by an endomysium
- Each muscle fibre is composed of bundles of myofibrils separated by the SR network
- The functional unit of the myofibril is called the sarcomere. There are many of these in each myofibril, being separated at the Z line
- The sarcomeres are formed from an arrangement of thick and thin filaments
- The thick and thin filaments are contractile proteins
- Thick filaments are formed from myosin
- Thin filaments are formed from actin, troponin and tropomysin

9. How does the action potential reaching the fibre finally give rise to a contraction?

The action potential brings about contraction through the process of *excitation-contraction coupling*:

- The action potential spreads out from the motor endplate through the T tubule system
- This causes the mobilisation of Ca^{2+} from the SR into the cytoplasm
- Ca^{2+} binds to Troponin C on the light chains
- This leads to the displacement of Tropomysin, so that myosin-binding sites are exposed on the actin chain
- Actin and myosin chains then cross-link onto one another
- Thick filaments of myosin slide on the actin thin filaments
- This final stage is made possible by the energy generated from the hydrolysis of adenosine

M

triphosphate (ATP) to adenosine diphosphate (ADP) by ATPase activity of the myosin head

10. Give some examples of where you might find smooth muscle in the body.

Examples include, the inner circular and outer longitudinal muscles in the wall of the gastrointestinal tract, muscle in the walls of blood vessels especially arterioles, detrusor muscle of the bladder, the myometrium of the uterus, and sphincter pupillae of the iris. There are numerous and varied examples.

11. How does the structure of smooth muscle differ from skeletal muscle?

There are several fundamental differences:

- Smooth muscle, as can be expected from such a wide distribution in the body, show great variability in the size and morphology of the fibres – reflecting the wide variation in tasks required in different systems

- Smooth muscle cells are often bunched into interweaving bundles of fibres bound together with collagen

- Gap junctions separate individual fusiform muscle cells. This type of connection causes a rapid transmission of excitation throughout the smooth cell population in an organ, e.g. during a coordinated contraction wave along a segment of bowel

- Actin and myosin filaments are not arranged as sarcomeres in smooth muscle. Instead, these filaments are irregularly arranged throughout the cell

- The SR is more poorly developed in smooth muscle

- T tubules are absent from smooth muscle

- Thin (actin) filaments are bound to 'dense' bodies which anchor them to the cell membrane

▼

12. How is contraction generated in smooth muscle?

- Contraction can be generated spontaneously by some types of smooth muscle cells, e.g. in the bowel wall. Like cardiac cells, such cells have unstable membrane potentials that decay spontaneously, producing contraction. Such spontaneous depolarisations that can be large enough to generate action potential are called *slow waves* and can be readily demonstrated in the bowel wall

[handwritten margin note: interstitial cells of Cajal. ↓ towards colon]

- Contraction may be generated by mechanical stretch of muscle fibres, e.g. in blood vessel walls. This is partly the basis for autoregulation of blood flow in the cerebral, coronary and renal vascular beds
- Stimulation is by neurotransmitter activation, e.g. acetylcholine-mediated activation of bronchial smooth muscle cell and bowel contractions

Note that unlike skeletal muscle, in smooth muscle, actin-myosin interaction and subsequent contraction occur following calcium-induced phosphorylation of myosin, mediated by the enzyme *myosin light-chain kinase*.

13. Which calcium-binding protein distinguishes smooth from skeletal muscle?

- In smooth muscle, the important Ca^{2+}-binding protein is *calmodulin*. This essentially permits phosphorylation of myosin filaments
- With skeletal muscle, the Ca^{2+}-binding protein is *troponin*, which is associated with thin (actin) filaments

M

MUSCLE I – SKELETAL AND SMOOTH MUSCLE

MUSCLE II – CARDIAC MUSCLE

1. Apart from the size of the fibres, what are the *structural* differences between skeletal and cardiac muscle?

Some structural differences:

- Cardiac cells are *mononuclear*, skeletal muscle cells are *multinuclear*

- The cardiac cell (myocyte) nucleus is centrally located, but peripherally located for skeletal cells

- Cardiac muscle fibres are branched, unlike skeletal fibres

- Cardiac cells are connected to one another by intercalated disks. Gap junctions at these discs allow excitation to pass from one cell to another. Therefore, cardiac myocytes contract as a *syncitium*

- The T tubule system (which spreads the action potential) is larger in cardiac muscle

- In cardiac muscle, such T tubules are located at the Z line. In skeletal muscle, it is located at the junction of the A and I bands

2. List some *functional* differences between skeletal and cardiac muscle.

- Skeletal muscle is voluntary

- Cardiac muscle contracts spontaneously (myogenic)

- In skeletal muscle, Ca^{2+} is released from the SR following spread of depolarisation through the T tubule network

- With cardiac muscle, Ca^{2+}-release from the SR is triggered by Ca^{2+} that already been released by the SR, and by Ca^{2+} that has influxed through membrane voltage channels. This is called Ca^{2+}-*induced* Ca^{2+} *release*

▼

- Mechanical summation and tetanus do not occur with cardiac muscle because of the longer duration of cardiac action potential
- In the case of skeletal muscle, increases in force are generated by *recruitment* of motor units and *mechanical summation (see 'Skeletal muscle')*
- The force of cardiac muscle contraction is determined by the amount of intracellular Ca^{2+} generated. For example through the action of hormones
- Note than in both types of muscle, the initial fibre length at rest (preload) also determines the strength of contraction

3. Draw the action potential curve for the sino atrial (SA) node, and a ventricular myocyte. What is the ionic basis for the shape of the ventricular myocyte action potential?

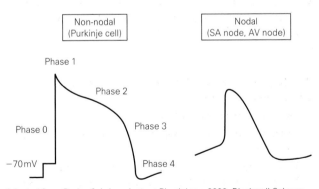

Adapted from Borley & Achan. Instant Physiology, 2000, Blackwell Science

The ionic fluxes that are responsible for myocyte activation may be divided into a number of phases according to their timing in relation to the curve of the

M

MUSCLE II – CARDIAC MUSCLE

action potential:

- *Phase 0:* Rapid depolarisation – when threshold is reached (around $-60\,mV$), voltage-gated Na^+-channels open, permitting the influx of Na^+.
- *Phase 1:* Partial repolarisation – this occurs following closure of the voltage-gated Na^+-channels
- *Phase 2:* Plateau phase – this may last 200–400 ms. Occurs due to open voltage-gated Ca^{2+} allowing a *slow* inward current of Ca^{2+} that sustains depolarisation. A persisting outward current of K^+ out that balances the influx of calcium ensures that the membrane potential keeps steady during this plateau phase
- *Phase 3:* Repolarisation following closure of the Ca^{2+}-channels, with continued outflow of K^+
- *Phase 4:* Pacemaker potential – spontaneous depolarisation due to the inherent instability of the membrane potential of cardiac myocytes (*see below*)

4. What is the significance of the 'plateau phase' of myocyte depolarisation?

The long plateau phase caused by the slow and sustained influx of Ca^{2+} has two important consequences on myocyte performance:

- Myocytes cannot be stimulated to produce tetanic contractions
- Myocytes are not fatigueable

5. Why do the pacemaker cells of the heart fire spontaneously?

Pacemaker cells of the SA and AV nodes have unstable membrane potentials that decay spontaneously to produce an action potential without having to be stimulated. Other myocytes do exhibit this inherent instability, but to a lesser extent than the pacemaker cells.

▼

This is unlike the 'standard' worker myocyte that has a relatively stable membrane. When the membrane potential of the pacemaker cell drifts to about $-40\,mV$ from a $-60\,mV$ starting point, voltage-gated Na^+-channels open up as the action potential is triggered.

This instability of the membrane potential is caused by the progressive reduction of the membrane's permeability to K^+. The resulting retention of intracellular K^+ coupled with a continued background inflow of Na^+ and Ca^{2+} leads to a progressive increase in the membrane potential until the action potential is triggered.

6. Define Starling's law of the heart.

This states the strength of contraction is proportional to the initial fibre length at rest, up to a point. This length-tension relationship can be seen in the graph below. This law applies at the individual fibre level as well as the macroscopic level *in vivo*.

7. Draw the Starling curve that illustrates this law, labelling the axes.

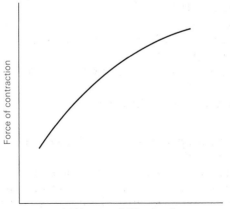

The x axis may also read "Ventricular end-diastolic pressure or end-diastolic volume"

8. What accounts for this relationship?

There are two main reasons why the strength of contraction increases with increased sarcomere length:

- At increased length, a greater number of actin filaments are exposed that can interact with the myosin heads. This also explains why skeletal muscle contraction increases with fibre stretch
- Length-dependent calcium sensitivity: through incompletely understood mechanisms, increasing the length of the sarcomere has been shown to improve the binding of calcium onto troponin C

9. How does digoxin affect the contractility of the myocyte? What is the mechanism of action?

Digoxin increases the inherent contractility of the myocyte, so that the strength of contraction is higher for any given sarcomere length.

This is a cardiac glycoside that inhibits the cardiac membrane Na^+-K^+ ATPase that normally pumps out Na^+ in exchange for K^+. Therefore, there is a rise in intracellular Na^+. This reduces the sodium gradient across the membrane, which in turn slows down the activity of the membrane Ca^{2+}-Na^+ pump. In doing so, there is intracellular accumulation of Ca^{2+}, leading to increased contractility.

10. What is the relationship between the strength of contraction and the rate of contraction? Why does this occur?

It is known that increasing the frequency of myocyte contraction also increases the strength of contraction. This is known as the '*Bowditch effect*'. It occurs because at higher frequencies of contraction, there is less time for intracellular Ca^{2+} to be pumped out of the cell between beats. Therefore, there is a progressive accumulation of intracellular calcium, leading to improved contractility.

11. Why is this relationship not seen in the heart *in vivo*?

This effect is not so clearly seen in the heart at the macroscopic level – in practise, increasing the heart rate in isolation serves only to reduce the time for diastolic filling, reducing the ventricular preload, and therefore the CO. This is why there is a fall in CO during tachyarrhythmias.

MUSCLE II – CARDIAC MUSCLE

NUTRITION: BASIC CONCEPTS

1. What are the body's sources of energy? How much energy does each supply?

- *Glucose:* provides $4.1 \, kcalg^{-1}$
- *Fat:* $9.3 \, kcalg^{-1}$
- *Protein:* $4.1 \, kcalg^{-1}$

2. What is meant by the *respiratory quotient*?

This is defined as the ratio of the volume of CO_2 produced to the volume of oxygen consumed from the oxidation of a given amount of nutrient. Values for the different energy sources are:

- *Carbohydrayte:* 1.0
- *Fat:* 0.7
- *Protein:* 0.8

3. What is the recommended daily intake for protein and nitrogen?

- *Protein:* $0.80 \, gkg^{-1}$
- *Nitrogen:* $0.15 \, gkg^{-1}$

4. What is an *essential* amino acid? How many are there, and give some examples?

These are amino acids that cannot be synthesised by the body and need to be ingested. There are 9 of them; leucine, isoleucine, lysine, methionine, phenylalanine, threonine, tryptophan, histidine and valine.

5. What are the main carbohydrates in the diet?

Dietary carbohydrate is composed mainly of the polysaccharide starch, some disaccharides such as sucrose and fructose and a small amount of lactose. Other important polysaccharides include cellulose, pectins and gums. These are not digested, and make up the roughage in the diet.

▼

6. In what form is fat stored in the body?

As triglycerides.

7. What are these composed of?

These consist largely of long chain saturated and unsaturated fatty acids (predominantly *palmitic, stearic* and *oleic* acids) that have been esterified to glycerol.

8. What is an *essential* fatty acid? Which ones are there, and why are they particularly important?

These are fatty acids that cannot be synthesised in the body. They are:

- Linoleic acid
- Linolenic acid
- Arachidonic acid

They are important for the synthesis of the eicosanoids, prostaglandins, leukotrienes and thromboxane.

9. In what form is dietary triglyceride that has just been absorbed transported in the body?

As chylomicrons.

10. What are the names of the vitamin B group? What deficiency diseases are associated with their deprivation?

- *Vitamin B_1 (Thiamine):* deficiency causes beri-beri or Wernicke's encephalopathy
- *Vitamin B_2 (Riboflavin):* deficiency leads to a syndrome of chelosis and glossitis
- *Vitamin B_3 (Niacin):* deficiency leads to pellagra
- *Biotin:* isolated deficiency is rare, but leads to enteritis and depressed immune function
- *Vitamin B_6 (Pyridoxine):* deficiency leads to peripheral neuropathy
- *Vitamin B_{12} (Cyanocobalamin):* deficiency leads to macrocytic anaemia

N

- Note that members of the vitamin B group are all water-soluble

11. Which are the fat-soluble vitamins and what functions do they have?

- *Vitamin A:* important for cell membrane stabilisation and retinal function
- *Vitamin D:* for calcium homeostasis, excitable cell function and bone mineralisation
- *Vitamin E:* free-radical scavenger and anti-oxidant
- *Vitamin K:* involved in the γ-carboxylation of glutamic acid residues of factors II, VII, IX and X during clotting

PANCREAS I – ENDOCRINE FUNCTIONS

1. What are the three cell types found in the pancreas' Islets of Langerhans, and what do they secrete?

- *α-cells:* secrete glucagon
- *β-cells:* secrete insulin
- *δ-cells:* secrete somatostatin

2. Other than insulin and glucagon, which other hormones may influence the serum [glucose]?

There are several, but the most important are:

- *Catacholamines:* epinephrine and norepinephrine
- *Glucocorticoids:* most important being cortisol
- *Somatotrophin:* a pituitary hormone

All of the above *increase* serum [glucose]. The only hormone that is known to *decrease* serum [glucose] is insulin.

3. What are the possible metabolic fates for glucose molecules in the body?

- *Glycolysis:* they may be metabolised by glycolysis and then to the tricarboxylic acid (TCA) cycle following the production of pyruvate
- *Storage:* as glycogen, through the process of glycogenesis. Most tissues of the body are able to do this
- *Protein glycosylation:* this is a normal process by which proteins are tagged with glucose molecules. This is by strict enzymatic control
- *Protein glycation:* this is where proteins are tagged with glucose in the presence of excess circulating [glucose]. It is not enzymatically controlled unlike the above example. An example of this is glycosylated haemoglobin
- *Sorbitol formation:* this occurs in various tissues when glucose enters the polyol pathway that ultimately leads to the formation of fructose from glucose

4. Where do the body's glucose molecules come from?

- *The diet*
- *Glycogenolysis:* following the breakdown of glycogen
- *Gluconeogenesis:* this is the generation of glucose from non-carbohydrate precursors

5. Give some examples of non-carbohydrate molecules that can be converted to glucose (by gluconeogenesis). Which tissues may generate glucose in this way?

Lactate, glycerol and some amino acids, such as alanine. The liver is the only tissue that can normally generate glucose in this way. However, during starvation, the kidneys may also perform gluconeogenesis.

6. What is the basic structure of insulin?

This is a protein hormone composed of an α and β sub-unit held together by disulphide bridges.

7. Give a list of some of the metabolic effects of insulin.

- *Carbohydrate*
  - Increases the uptake of glucose into various tissues
  - Stimulates glycogenesis in many tissues, but especially the liver
  - Stimulates hepatic generation of glucose-6-phosphate from glucose
- *Proteins*
  - Enhances the uptake of amino acids into peripheral tissues
  - Stimulates protein synthesis – for this reason, insulin can be regarded as one of the growth hormones
- *Fats*
  - Stimulates lipid uptake into cells
  - Enhances oxidation of lipids once inside cells

- Also causes fat deposition by stimulating lipogenesis in adipocytes and in the liver

• Note that, in addition, insulin increases the uptake of K^+ into cells, so has an influence on acid-base balance (*see 'Potassium balance'*)

8. How may ketoacidosis be triggered in diabetics?

• *The omission of insulin*
• *Infection*
• *Drug-induced:* such as cortisol, or thiazide diuretics, both of which lead to hyperglycaemia

9. What is the pathophysiology of ketosis?

Diabetes mellitus is a state akin to starvation. There is plenty of circulating glucose, but since there is a lack of insulin, the circulating glucose cannot be taken into the cell to be utilised. This leads to increased lipolysis and increased FFA production. Ketone bodies represent readily transportable fatty acids that can be utilised by organs such as the heart and brain. When there is a lack of glucose, improper utilisation of components of the citric acid cycle leads to a continued build up of ketones, leading to metabolic acidosis. The three ketone bodies: *acetone, acetoacetate* and *β-hydroxybutyrate.*

10. You are asked to examine a patient with chronic diabetes mellitus. What may you find on examination?

On examining the skin:

• Necobiosis lipoidica diabeticorum: seen as red-yellow plaques, usually found on the shin. They may ulcerate
• Leg ulcers
• Areas of fat atrophy where insulin is injected
• Skin infections: cellulites, carbuncles, boils or candidiasis

▼ 113

On examining the eyes:
- Diabetic retinopathy on fundal examination
- Cataracts

Features of peripheral vascular disease, with ulceration: there may be evidence of limb amputation, or gangrene.

On neurological examination:
- Presence of a peripheral Charcot's joint
- Features of diabetic neuropathy, such as reduced sensation and dorsal column function

Features of chronic renal failure: such as skin pigmentation, hypertension, presence of an iatrogenic peripheral arterial fistula in the wrist (for vascular access during haemodialysis).

PANCREAS II – EXOCRINE FUNCTIONS

1. What type of gland is the pancreas?

It is a mixed endocrine and exocrine gland.

2. Microscopically, which other organ does the exocrine component of the pancreas resemble?

The parotid salivary gland. The functional unit of the exocrine pancreas is the acinus. Each acinus consists of a group of polygonal acinar cells that lead into a system of secretory ducts.

3. Roughly, what is the daily volume of pancreatic juice produced?

1–1.5 l daily.

4. What is the juice basically composed of?

There are two main components to the juice:

- *An aqueous component:* containing water, bicarbonate and other ions
- *An enzymatic component:* containing digestive enzymes

5. What are the most important ions found in the secretions of the exocrine pancreas?

- HCO_3^-: at basal secretion, pancreatic juice contains more than twice the concentration of bicarbonate ions as the plasma
- Cl^-: at basal secretion, this is slightly at lower concentration than the plasma
- Na^+: similar concentration to the plasma
- K^+: similar concentration to the plasma
- *Note that it has a high pH*

▼ 115

P

6. Below is a graph showing the variation in the concentration of pancreatic juice ions during a certain circumstance. What is this circumstance that should be labelled on the x-axis?

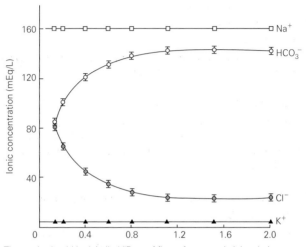

The x-axis should be labelled "Rare of flow of pancreatic juice during pancreatic stimulation"

Adapted from Berne RM, Levy MN. Principles of Physiology, 3rd edition, 2000, with permission from Elsevier

7. Why is there a reciprocal relationship between bicarbonate and chloride ions?

This is because the two ions are exchanges at the acinar cell membrane, so that chloride is absorbed into the cell from the lumen of the ducts in exchange for increased bicarbonate output into the secretions.

8. List the enzymes secreted by the pancreas. Which molecules are they responsible for the digestion of?

- *Proteases*
  - Trypsinogen
  - Chymotrypsinogen

▼

- ■ Procarboxypeptidase
- ■ Proelastase
- *Lipolytic*
  - ■ Lipase
  - ■ Phospholipase A_2
- *Starch digestion:*
  - ■ α-amylase

Note that the proteases are secreted as the *inactive zymogen* forms that require activation.

9. How are they activated?

Trypsinogen is activated by enteropeptidase (also called enterokinase) that is secreted by the mucosa of the duodenum. The trypsin released is then able to activate the other enzymes.

10. Which factors stimulate pancreatic secretion?

- *Vagal stimulation*
- *Secretin:* a hormone produced by the duodenal mucosa following the appearance of acid. Predominantly stimulates the aqueous component
- *CCK:* released from the duodenum following the appearance of fatty food
- *Gastrin:* causes less pronounced stimulation

11. Taking all of this into account, outline the effects of a total pancreatectomy.

- *Development of diabetes mellitus*
- *Reduced fat absorption:* leading to steatorrhoea together with malabsorption of the fat-soluble vitamins A, D, E, and K
- *Reduced protein absorption:* leading to a negative nitrogen balance
- *Reduced absorption of Fe^+ and Ca^{2+}:* this is due to the loss of alkalinisation of the chyme from the stomach that normally promotes the absorption of these

ions. Therefore leads to iron-deficiency anaemia and osteoporosis/rickets

12. Can you think of why those who have been rendered diabetic by pancreatectomy are very sensitive to exogenous insulin therapy?

This is because there is also an absolute lack of glucagon (also secreted by the pancreatic islets). This hormone normally counteracts insulin and places a negative feedback on its metabolic effects.

POTASSIUM BALANCE

P

1. What is the normal range for serum potassium?

3.5–5.0 mmol^{-1}.

2. What is the distribution of potassium in the body?

About 98% of the body's potassium is intracellular. Thus, the intracellular concentration is ~150 mmol^{-1} compared to the serum concentration of ~4 mmol^{-1}.

3. Which factors are responsible for the regulation of serum potassium?

- *Dietary intake:* a typical 'Western' diet contains 20–100 mmol of potassium daily
- *Aldosterone:* a steroid hormone of the adrenal cortex. Stimulates absorption of sodium in the DCT of the kidney, and several other organs, at the expense of potassium loss through active exchange at the cell membrane
- *Acid-base balance:* potassium and H$^+$ are exchanged at the cell membrane, so that an increase of one ion leads to increased exchange with the other, e.g. acidosis leads to hyperkalaemia and vice versa. Such membrane exchange occurs in the kidney tubules as well as other cells
- *Tubular fluid flow rate:* increased flow leads to potassium loss – this is one way in which diuretics promote hypokalaemia
- *Insulin:* stimulates potassium intake into cells, reducing the serum level

4. Give some causes of hyperkalaemia.

- *Artefact:* e.g. haemolysis in the blood bottle
- *Iatrogenic:* excess external administration
- *Following internal redistribution:*
  - *Between intracellular fluid (ICF) and ECF* due to injury, e.g. crush injury, burns, intravascular haemolysis
  - *Reduced cellular uptake:* diabetes mellitus, acidosis

- *Decreased excretion:*
  - *Renal:* renal failure, potassium-sparing diuretics
  - *Adrenal origin:* Addison's disease
  - *Mineralocorticoid resistance:* systemic lupus erythematosus (SLE), chronic interstitial nephritis

5. Which ECG changes may you see with hyperkalaemia?

- Tall and tented T-waves
- Small P-waves
- Wide QRS complex

6. Give some causes of hypokalaemia.

- *Artefact:* e.g. drip-arm sampling
- *Decreased oral intake*
- *Internal re-distribution:*
  - *Between ECF and ICF:* alkalosis, excess insulin (iatrogenic, insulinoma)
- *Loss from the body:*
  - *GIT losses:* vomiting, diarrhoea, mucin-secreting colonic adenoma, entero-cutaneous fistula
  - *Renal loses:* Conn's syndrome, use of loop and thiazide diuretics

7. Which ECG changes might you see?

- Small or inverted T-waves
- Prolonged PR-interval
- S–T segment depression

PROXIMAL TUBULE AND LOOP OF HENLE

1. What is the principle function of the proximal convoluted tubule (PCT)?

This structure is the kidney's major site for reabsorption of solutes – in fact, 70% of filtered solutes are reabsorbed at the PCT.

2. What kinds of solute?

The most important are sodium, chloride and potassium ions. In addition, nearly all of the glucose and amino acids filtered by the glomerulus are reabsorbed here.

The first half of the PCT also absorbs phosphate and lactate.

3. Which membrane pump system is key to the PCT reabsorptive abilities?

The Na^+-K^+ ATPase pump.

4. What are the basic functions of the loop of Henle?

- *Solute reabsorption:* about 20% of filtered sodium, chloride and potassium ions are absorbed in the *thick ascending limb* of Henle
- *Water reabsorption:* about 20% of filtered water is absorbed at the *thin descending limb* of Henle
- *Formation of the counter current multiplication system:* this is an efficient way of concentrating the urine over a relatively short distance along the nephron with minimal energy expenditure

5. Why there is no water reabsorption at the ascending limb of Henle?

This portion of the loop of Henle is impermeable to water.

6. What is the basic function of the DCT and collecting duct?

- *Reabsorption of solute:* about 12% of filtered sodium and potassium are absorbed here
- *Secretion:* variable amounts of potassium and protons are secreted here
- *Reabsorption of water:* this occurs only at the most distal portions of the DCT and collecting duct, since the more proximal areas are impermeable to water

7. What is one of the most important factors regulating the reabsorption of solutes and water across the PCT and loop of Henle?

The Starling forces *(see Microcirculation I).*

8. Which hormone plays a central role in the control of water excretion?

ADH (also known as arginine vasopressin).

9. Where is this hormone produced?

In the posterior pituitary gland.

10. How does the body monitor changes in the plasma osmolality?

By the activity of osmoreceptors located in the hypo-thalamus.

11. Thus, what are the two most important factors in controlling the release of ADH?

- *Increased plasma osmolality:* water loss leads to an increase in the plasma [Na^+], which increases the plasma osmolality
- *Decrease in the effective circulating volume:* this triggers activity in vascular baroreceptors

12. Once released, what is the effect of ADH on the kidney?

This leads to an increase in the reabsorption of solute-free water by the collecting duct.

Also leads to NaCl reabsorption by the *thick ascending limb* of Henle. By increasing the concentration of the interstitium around the loop of Henle, this enhances the nephron's ability to reabsorb water.

13. Draw a simplified diagram of the loop of Henle when ADH secretion is maximal during a period of dehydration. What is happening?

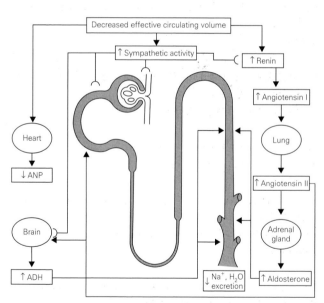

From Koeppen BE, Stanton BA. Renal Physiology, 1992, London, with permission from Elsevier

1. Fluid enters the descending limb of Henle that is isotonic with the plasma. The tubular fluid that leaves the PCT is always isotonic with the plasma

2. The descending limb of Henle is permeable to water (and only slightly permeable to salt and urea. Therefore, water is progressively absorbed down the limb, becoming more and more concentrated (up to $1,200\,\text{mOsmol}^{-1}$)

3. The ascending limb of Henle is impermeable to water, but permeable to sodium chloride. There is passive diffusion of NaCl down its concentration gradient, when travelling up the limb. This dilutes the tubular fluid

4. When the thick ascending limb is reached, NaCl is actively pumped out, further diluting the tubular fluid. *ADH increases the pumping of NaCl into the interstitium*

5. By the time that the tubular fluid reaches the collecting duct, it is hypotonic compared to the interstitium. Therefore, in the presence of ADH (which increases the water-permeability of the collecting duct), water is rapidly reabsorbed

6. By the time that urine is excreted, it has a very high osmolality (up to $1,200\,\text{mOsmol}^{-1}$)

PULMONARY BLOOD FLOW

1. If the normal CO at rest is said to be 5–6 Lmin^{-1}, what is the output of the right side of the heart?

This is also 5–6 Lmin^{-1} since under normal circumstances; the outputs of both sides of the heart are the same.

2. Give a normal value for the pulmonary artery pressure (PAP).

$$\frac{25}{8} \text{ mmHg.}$$

3. Why is this so much lower than the systemic arterial pressure?

The principle reason is that the pulmonary vascular resistance is only about *one tenth* of the systemic vascular resistance.

4. Define the PVR. Give the normal range.

This is defined by the equation:

$$PVR = \frac{PAP - CVP}{CO} \times 80$$

where PAP = mean PA pressure; CVP = central venous pressure; CO = cardiac output

The normal range is 150–250 dynes-sec/cm^5. Note that if not multiplying by 80, then the calculated figure for the resistance is given in *Wood* units.

5. Below is a graph showing the relationship of the PVR to increasing pulmonary arterial and venous

P

pressures. Briefly, what does this show, and why does this occur?

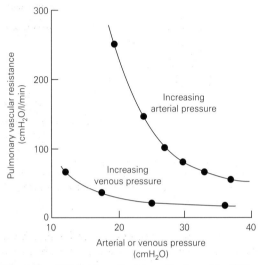

From West JB. Respiratory Physiology: The Essentials, 1989, Lippincott, Williams & Wilkins

- This shows that the PVR falls with rising pulmonary and venous pressures
- This occurs because of distension of the thin-walled pulmonary vessels when engorged with blood following a pressure rise. This distension leads to an overall fall in the PVR. Also, the recruitment of previously empty pulmonary vessels adds further to a fall in the PVR. The concepts of pulmonary vascular distension and recruitment can be pictorially seen below, the effects of both being to drop the PVR

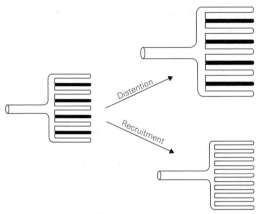

Increased pulmonary blood flow can lead either to
distension of pulmonary vessels, or to recruitment of collapsed vessels

From NMS: Physiology, 4th edition, Bullock, Boyle & Wang, 2001,
Lippincott, Williams & Wilkins

**6. Below is a graph showing the relationship between
the PVR and the lung volume at constant intra-alveolar
pressure. Again, what does this show, and what is the
explanation?**

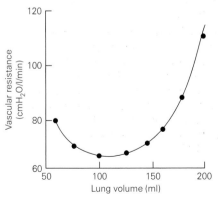

From West JB. Respiratory Physiology: The Essentials, 1989,
Lippincott, Williams & Wilkins

- This shows that at very low lung volumes, the PVR is relatively high, but soon falls following distension of the lungs. After this initial fall, with increasing volumes, the PVR rises again. This rise in the PVR following the initial dip is virtually exponential

- Much of these changes can be explained in terms of the elastic forces generated by the collagen and elastin of the lung parenchyma *(see 'Mechanics of breathing IV')*. At increasing lung volumes, the elastic recoil forces of the lung increase. This produces a circumferential *radial traction* force that pulls small airways (i.e. those without cartilaginous walls) and blood vessels open; thus reducing their resistance to the flow of air and blood respectively

- At very small lung volumes, due to little radial traction, pulmonary vessels are collapsed. This has the effect of increasing the overall PVR

- As the lung expands, radial traction forces on the blood vessels increase, increasing their calibre. This causes a progressive fall in the PVR

- At increasing volumes, radial traction *overstretches* the pulmonary vessels, reducing their calibre. Thus, once again, the PVR rises, and blood flow falls

7. Taking the above into account, summarise the factors controlling the PVR, and hence the pulmonary blood flow.

- *Pulmonary arterial and venous pressure*
- *Lung volume*
- *Pulmonary vascular smooth muscle tone:* this is affected by various mediators, such as the catacholamines, histamine, 5-HT, and arachidonic acid metabolites
- *Hypoxia:* this also has an effect on the smooth muscle tone, but is listed separately due to its importance. This leads to pulmonary vasoconstriction, with an increase in the PVR. The result of this is to improve the ventilation-perfusion ratio in the lung in the face of a fall in the PaO_2.

It can therefore be considered to be a defence mechanism against the deleterious effects of hypoxia, e.g. in situations of COPD. However, chronic hypoxia, can lead to irreversible pulmonary hypertension with progressive right heart failure (cor pulmonale). *(See also 'Ventilation-perfusion relationships in the lung'.)*

8. Nitric oxide (NO) is the main method by which many of these mediators act. It is also often used in the management of pulmonary hypertension in the critically ill. What is its mode of action?

- It has a very short duration of action, and functions through stimulation of intracellular Guanylate cyclase, which produces cGMP from GTP. This in turn stimulates cGMP-dependant protein kinases that are involved in causing vessel wall smooth muscle cell relaxation
- Bradykinin and 5-HT are examples of mediators that act through NO

9. Under normal circumstances, how is the blood flow in the lungs distributed?

- In the standing position, the lowest parts of the lungs receive the greatest blood flow. In fact, a linear decrease in the blood flow distribution can be seen from apex to base
- This is because the hydrostatic pressure of the most dependent portions is greater

10. How does this alter with exercise?

During mild exercise, the blood flow to the upper and lower portions of the lung increases, but the overall distribution of the flow is more even than during rest.

RENAL BLOOD FLOW (RBF)

R

1. What percentage of the CO do the kidneys receive?

20–25%, so that the RBF is 1.0–1.2 L min^{-1}.

2. Below is a graph showing the variation of the RBF with the arterial pressure. What does this show?

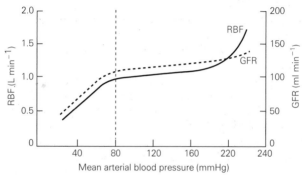

Mean arterial blood pressure (mmHg)

From Lecture Notes on Human Physiology, 3rd edition, Bray, Cragg, Macknight, Mills & Taylor, 1994, Oxford, Blackwell Science

This graph shows that the RBF, like many specialised vascular beds, is controlled largely by *autoregulation.* Thus, between mean arterial pressures of 80–180 mmHg, RBF is fairly constant, at about 1.2 L min^{-1}.

3. How is this achieved?

There are two main theories to explain how renal autoregulation of blood flow occurs:

- *Myogenic mechanism:* an increase in renal vascular wall tension that occurs following a sudden rise in arterial pressure stimulates mural smooth muscle cells to contract, causing vasoconstriction. This reduces the RBF in the face of rising arterial pressures. Most of this myogenic response occurs in the afferent arteriole

- *Tubuloglomerular feedback:* alterations in the flow of blood that occurs with alterations in the arterial pressure leads to stimulation of the juxtaglomerular apparatus. This leads to a poorly defined feedback loop that results in changes of the RBF to the baseline level

4. Name some other factors that are important for the control of RBF.

- *SNS:* this controls the tone of the afferent and efferent arteriole. By stimulation of α_1-adrenoceptors there is vasoconstriction and reduction of blood flow
- *Angiotensin II:* as part of the control by the renin-, angiotensin-aldosterone system. This hormone stimulates vasoconstriction, leading to a reduction of the RBF and GFR
- *Local mediators:* such as PGE_2 and PGI_2, both of which cause arteriolar vasoconstriction

5. Which agent has traditionally been used to measure the RBF?

The organic acid, *para-aminohippuric acid* (PAH).

6. Which physiologic properties make it ideal for the measurement of the RBF?

PAH in the circulation is completely eliminated through the processes of filtration and secretion by the tubules, so that there is none found in the renal vein following passage through the kidneys. Therefore, in effect, the rate of clearance of PAH from the circulation in equal to the renal plasma flow (RPF). This can be seen below:

$$RPF = \frac{U_{PAH} \cdot V}{P_{PAH}}$$

R

where U_{PAH} = Urine PAH concentration; P_{PAH} = Plasma PAH concentration.

7. How can the RBF be calculated from the RPF?

$$RBF = \frac{\cancel{RBF} \, RPF}{1 - HCT}$$

where RPF = renal plasma flow; HCT = haematocrit.

RESPIRATORY FUNCTION TESTS

1. Draw a typical spirometry tracing, and label the various volumes that the waveforms represent.

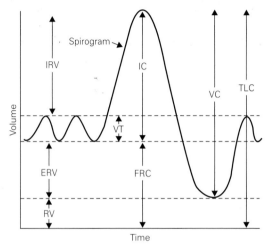

From NMS: Physiology, 4th edition. Bullock, Boyle & Wang, 2001, Lippincott, Williams & Wilkins

2. Which of the volumes and capacities may be measured directly?

Note that the 'capacities' are derived by adding 'volumes' together. The following can be measured directly:

- Tidal volume (TV)
- Inspiratory reserve volume (IRV)
- Expiratory reserve volume (ERV)
- Inspiratory capacity (IC) = (TV + IRV)
- Vital capacity (VC) = (IRV + TV + ERV)

3. Then, which must be calculated by other sources?

- Residual volume (RV)

- FRC = (RV + ERV)
- Total lung volume (TLV) = (VC + RV)

4. Give some typical values for the TV, IRV and ERV.

- *TV:* 500 ml, or 7 mlkg^{-1}
- *IRV:* defined as the volume that can be inspired above the TV. Typically 3.0 L
- *ERV:* the volume of gas that can be expired after a quiet expiration. Typically 1.3 L

5. Define RV.

This is the volume that remains in the lung following maximal expiration, and may only be measured using the same method as the FRC (see below). The normal value is around 1.2–1.5 L.

6. Define FRC. How may it be measured?

This is defined as the sum of the RV and the ERV. It represents the volume of gas left in the lung at the end of a quiet expiration.

There are three main methods for its measurement:

- *Gas dilution method:* using helium placed within the spirometer. The subject breathes through the system starting at the end of a quiet expiration. Helium is not absorbed by the blood but distributed throughout the lungs. The concentration of helium expired at the end of equilibration can be used to calculate the FRC

  Total amount of helium = Volume of gas in spirometer × initial concentration of helium = Helium concentration at equilibration × (volume of spirometer + FRC)

- *Nitrogen washout:* subject breathes pure oxygen from the end point of a quiet expiration. By analysing the changes in the concentration of nitrogen, the FRC may be calculated

▼

- *Plethysmography:* uses an airtight chamber to measure the total volume of gas in the lungs

7. What is the normal range for the FRC? What factors may cause it to increase or decrease?

The normal range is 2.5–3.0 L.

It may be decreased by:
- Supine position
- Any restrictive lung disease
- Pregnancy
- Following abdominal surgery
- Following anaesthesia

It may be increased by continuous positive airway pressure (CPAP) and gaseous retention of obstructive lung diseases.

8. What is the 'effective' TV?

This is defined as the TV−anatomic dead space, and represents the volume of inspired air that reaches the alveoli.

9. What is the definition of 'dead space'?

This is the volume of inspired air that is not involved in gas exchange.

10. What types of dead space volume do you know?

There are three types of dead space:
- *Anatomic dead space:* formed by the gas conduction parts of the airway that are not involved in gas exchange, such as the mouth, nasal cavity, pharynx, trachea and upper bronchial airways. Measured using *Fowler's method*
- *Alveolar dead space:* composed of those alveoli that are being ventilated but not perfused. They are therefore, in effect, not contributing to gas exchange

R

- *Physiologic dead space:* this is the sum of the two volumes above. The normal value is $2-3\,ml\,kg^{-1}$ measured using *Bohr's method*

SMALL INTESTINE

1. What is the main function of the small intestine?

This is the principle site for the absorption of carbohydrate, lipid, proteins, water, electrolytes, vitamins and essential minerals.

2. What is the transit time for chyme to pass through the small bowel?

2–4 h.

3. What are the three main types of small bowel motion seen after a meal?

- *Peristalsis:* in common with the rest of the gut
- *Segmentation:* more frequent than the above, occurring about 8 times per minute in the ileum, lasting for several seconds. Involves localised contraction of 1–2 cm of bowel that leads to the propulsion of chyme in both directions. Important for mixing chyme with the digestive juices
- *Pendular movements:* longitudinal muscle contractions lead to movement of the bowel wall over luminal contents. Also important for mixing

4. How does the motility differ when the small bowel is empty of contents?

During fasting, a *migrating motor complex* spreads from the duodenum to the ileocaecal junction. This contractile wave helps to clear the small bowel of any remaining contents.

5. What is the composition of small bowel secretions?

This is made up of mucous, water and NaCl, predominantly.

6. What is the output of this daily?

1,500 mL per day.

7. How does this compare to the rest of the gut?

The daily volume of gut secretions in (mL per day) may be summarised:

- *Saliva:* 1,500
- *Gastric:* 2,000
- *Bile:* 500
- *Pancreatic:* 1,500
- *Small intestine:* 1,500

8. How much water does the small bowel absorb per day?

Assuming that oral intake is 2,000 mL daily, the small bowel absorbs about 8,500 mL of water daily. The colon, about 400 mL daily. This leaves around 100 mL excreted in the faeces per day.

9. What are the effects of terminal ilectomy?

- *Loss of bile salt re-uptake:* this alters the colonic flora and changes the consistency of stools. There is also increased bile salt manufacture by the liver in response to reduced uptake, increasing the incidence of gallstones
- *Decreased Vitamin B_{12} uptake:* producing macrocytic anaemia
- *Reduced water absorption:* this is one of the important functions of the terminal ileum. This can lead to loose and frequent stools
- *Reduced uptake of γ-globulin:* the terminal ileum is full of lymphatic tissue, and there is some re-uptake of immunoglobulin. Loss of this tissue may affect local gut immune surveillance

SODIUM BALANCE

S

1. What is the major distribution of sodium in the body?

Sodium is the major extracellular cation of the body:

- 50% is found in the ECF
- 45% found in the bone
- 5% in the intracellular compartment
- Note that 70% of this ion is found in a readily-exchangeable form

2. What is the major physiological role for this ion?

This is the ion that generates the greatest osmotic force. For this reason, it is vital for the internal water balance between the intracellular and extracellular spaces. The osmolality that it generates also influences the control of the ECF volume that is under renal control.

This osmotic role occurs because this ion is so abundant in the body.

3. What is the daily sodium requirement?

$1 \, \mathrm{mmol\,kg^{-1}}$ per day.

4. Give some causes for hyponatraemia.

- *Water excess*
  - *Increased intake:* polydipsia, iatrogenic, e.g. TURP syndrome, excess administration of dextrose
  - *Water retention:* syndrome of inappropriate ADH (SIADH)
  - *Retention of water (with a bit of salt):* nephrotic syndrome, cardiac failure, hepatic failure
- *Water loss (with greater sodium loss)*
  - *Renal losses:* diuretics, Addison's disease
  - *Gut losses:* diarrhoea, vomiting

- *Pseudohyponatraemia:* measuring the sodium inaccurately in the presence of hyperlipidaemia

5. What does the *inappropriate* in SIADH refer to?

In SIADH, there is an excessive and pathological retention of water in the absence of renal, adrenal or thyroid disease. The 'inappropriate' refers to the fact that the urine osmolality is inappropriately high in relation to the plasma osmolality.

6. Which conditions may trigger the SIADH?

- *Lung pathology:* pneumonia, lung abscess and TB
- *Malignancy:* small cell carcinoma of the lung, brain tumours, prostatic carcinoma
- *Other intra-cranial pathology:* head injury, meningitis
- *Alcohol withdrawal*

7. What are the causes of hypernatraemia?

- *Water loss*
  - Diabetes insipidus
  - Insufficient intake or administration
  - Osmotic diuresis, e.g. hyperglycaemia
- *Excess sodium over water*
  - Conn's or Cushing's syndrome
  - Excess hypertonic saline

8. What is diabetes insipidus?

This is a syndrome of polyuria with hypernatraemia and dehydration with compensatory polydipsia caused by an insensitivity to (nephrogenic form) or deficiency of (cranial form) ADH. Characteristically, fluid deprivation fails to concentrate the urine.

SODIUM AND WATER BALANCE

1. What are the main fluid compartments of the body, and what are their volumes?
- *Intracellular space:* 28 L
- *Extracellular space:* 14 L
  - *Plasma:* 3 L
  - *Interstitium:* 10 L
  - *Transcellular space:* 1 L

Therefore, the total body water is ~42 L.

2. What are the two main systems of water balance in the body, and what important feature do they have in common?
- *Internal water balance:* this system governs water balance between the intracellular and extracellular compartments. It relies on the balance between the osmolalities of the two compartments
- *External water balance:* this governs the extracellular fluid volume. The point of control is at the plasma-interstitial, and plasma-renal tubule interfaces. The *Starling forces* are important in this system of control
- Both systems are reliant on sodium balance since this is the most osmotically influential ion. It follows that since sodium determines plasma osmolality, it also plays an important role in regulation of the extracellular circulating volume

3. List the hormones that are important in maintaining the ECF volume.
- *ADH:* also known as arginine vasopressin. Produced by the posterior pituitary gland, and increases free water absorption by the collecting duct
- *Atrial naturetic peptide:* produced by the cardiac atria when distended. This has the opposite effect to ADH, but also increases sodium excretion

- *Hormones of the R-A-A axis:* broadly speaking, these have a long-term effect on the control of the circulating volume and arterial pressure
- *Glucocorticoids:* these increase sodium and water reabsorption
- *Catacholamines:* through altering the arterial pressure, they stimulate the release of the hormones of the R-A-A system. These are secreted by renal sympathetic nerves when there is a fall in the renal perfusion pressure

4. How does the body monitor the ECF volume?

Through a series of receptors that monitor the intravascular volumes and pressures.

5. Where in the body are these located?

- *Low-pressure receptors:* baroreceptors are located in the walls of the cardiac atria and pulmonary vessels, and they respond to distension that occurs with an increase in the circulating volume
- *High-pressure volume receptors:* these are baroreceptors located in the aortic arch, carotid sinus and afferent arteriole of the kidney. Also there is the *juxtaglomerular apparatus* of the kidney

6. What is the juxtaglomerular apparatus composed of?

This is formed from three components:

- *The macula densa:* of the thick ascending limb
- *Granular cells of the afferent and efferent arterioles*
- *Mesangial cells:* these act as antigen-presenting cells

7. Why is this structure so important to the control of the circulating volume and sodium balance?

The granular cells of this apparatus produce *renin*, which goes on to initiate the R-A-A cascade.

▼

8. Under what conditions is the R-A-A system stimulated?

The trigger to the release of renin by the juxtaglomerular apparatus is three fold:

- *Fall of renal perfusion pressure:* this is principally detected by the baroreceptors of the afferent arterioles
- *Activation of the SNS:* this occurs when there is a fall in the arterial pressure
- *Reduced sodium delivery to the macula densa:* this also occurs when there is a fall in the renal perfusion pressure

Below is a summary of the components of the R-A-A system

S

SODIUM AND WATER BALANCE

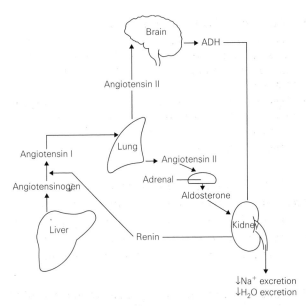

From Koeppen BE, Stanton BA. Renal Physiology, 1992, London, with permission from Elsevier

9. What is the effect of activation of this system?

- Stimulation of aldosterone release by the adrenal cortex, this increases sodium and water reabsorption, helping to maintain the arterial pressure

- Angiotensin causes vasoconstriction, increasing the peripheral vascular resistance, and so the arterial pressure. Resulting vasoconstriction also reduces the GFR at a time when water has to be conserved

- Stimulation of ADH secretion by the posterior pituitary, which leads to increased solute-free water reabsorption and thirst

- Enhanced NaCl reabsorption by the PCT

STARVATION

S

1. What is the difference between starvation, fasting and cachexia?

- *Starvation* is a chronic state resulting from inadequate intake of energy
- *Fasting* is a state of energy deprivation lasting no more than several days
- *Cachexia* is the state resulting from a chronic deprivation of energy and nutrients irrespective of the adequacy of intake, e.g. in malignant cachexia, there is protein and energy malnutrition even when there is adequate intake of food

2. What is the basic difference between *marasmus* and *kwashiorkor*?

- *Marasmus* is characterised by inadequacy of all nutrients and energy sources
- *Kwashiokor* is characterised by a lack of protein, but there is some intake of energy sources

3. During a period of fasting, from which source does the body obtain glucose?

From glycogen, found most abundantly in the liver and skeletal muscle.

4. How long does this supply last?

About 24 h.

5. When this supply is exhausted, why doesn't the body become hypoglycaemic?

Because, through gluconeogenesis, the liver is able to convert some molecules into glucose.

6. What are the substrates for gluconeogenesis?

- *Glycerol:* which is released from the breakdown of triglycerides
- *Amino acids:* from the so-called glucogenic amino acids, such as alanine

S

- *Lactate:* production of which is increased following fasting and starvation

7. What is the result of fasting on the body's store of protein and fat?

- In the early stages of fasting, because of the requirements for gluconeogenesis, there is a rapid breakdown of muscle to release amino acid, which is transported to the liver for conversion to glucose. This breakdown of muscle slows down the longer starvation proceeds
- Adipose tissue is continually broken down into free fatty acids and glycerol. This mobilisation of the adipose tissue becomes relatively more important the longer the period of starvation goes on

8. Summarise briefly the differences between fasting and prolonged starvation, in terms of the biochemical adaptation.

- During starvation, relatively more adipose tissue is being mobilised
- Also, there is relatively less muscle protein mobilisation
- There is increased generation of ketone bodies as a source of energy during starvation

9. Name the ketone bodies.

- Acetone
- Acetoacetate
- β-hydroxybutyrate

10. Which organ is particularly reliant on ketones during starvation?

The brain. This organ is usually heavily dependant on glucose as its energy source, but during starvation, adapts to using ketones.

▼

11. How else does the body adapt to starvation?

There is a general reduction of energy requirement, which is partly due to a reduction in the BMR brought on through a fall in the secretion of tri-iodothyronine by the thyroid, and reduced peripheral conversion of T_4.

12. Which hormones are the most important for the mediation of the body's adaptation to starvation?

- *Glucocorticoids:* these act to increase serum [glucose]
- *Catacholamines:* these cause a temporary increase in the serum [glucose]
- *Glucagon*
- *Thyroid hormone:* as mentioned above
- *Insulin:* a lack of the effects of this hormone triggers the adaptive response

S

STOMACH I

1. What are gastric secretions composed of?

These are both *exocrine* and *endocrine* in nature:

- *Water*
- *Mucus*
- *Ions:* notably hydrochloric acid and bicarbonate
- *Pepsinogen:* enzyme precursor for protein digestion
- *Intrinsic factor:* for the absorption of vitamin B_{12}
- *Hormones:* gastrin is the main one, also histamine from regional mast cells

2. Which gastric cells are involved in these secretions?

Note that these cells are located within the gastric glands, the entrance to which is seen on the surface as *gastric pits:*

- *Parietal cells:* secretion of HCl *and* intrinsic factor. Most frequently in the glands of the fundus
- *Chief cells:* secreting pepsinogen, the precursor of pepsin
- *Mucous cells:* most frequently found in the necks of the gastric glands of the pylorus
- *G-cells:* found in the glands of the pylorus and they secrete the hormone gastrin

3. Why does the stomach secrete acid?

There are three main reasons:

- HCl has some proteolytic activity
- By reducing the gastric pH to 2, it provides the ideal environment for the gastric enzyme pepsin
- Has antibacterial properties and prevents colonisation

4. What is the volume of gastric secretion daily?

1–1.5 L per day.

5. How is hydrochloric acid produced by the parietal cell?

This may be summarised in the diagram below:

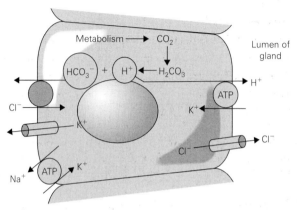

From Berne RM, Levy MN. Principles of Physiology, 3rd edition, 2000, London, with permission from Elsevier

- There is the initial active transport of K^+ and Cl^- into the cell
- H^+ that is generated from CO_2 dissolving into the cytoplasm is actively exchanged with K^+ at the H^+-K^+ ATPase. The H^+ enters the gastric lumen
- The HCO_3^- generated through dissociation of H_2CO_3 diffuses back into the plasma in exchange for Cl^-
- Chloride now enters the gastric lumen

6. How is the production of gastric acid controlled?

HCl secretion is stimulated by:

- *ACh:* from parasympathetic vagal neurones that innervate the parietal cells directly
- *Gastrin:* produced by pyloric G-cells

- *Histamine:* produced by mast cells. This stimulates the parietal cells directly and also potentiates parietal cell stimulation by gastrin and neuronal stimulation

HCl secretion is inhibited by:

- *Somatostatin:* from cells in the enteric nervous system
- *Secretin:* produced by the duodenum and inhibits gastrin release
- *CCK:* also inhibits gastrin release

7. Can you name some drugs that inhibit gastric acid secretion?

- *Omeprazole:* one of the proton-pump (H^+-K^+ ATPase) inhibitors
- *Cimetidine, ranitidine:* anti histamines that prevent mast cell stimulation of parietal cells
- *Acetazolamide:* inhibits the enzyme *carbonic anhydrase,* which catalyses the reaction that sees to HCO_3^- generation within the parietal cell

8. How does the stomach protect itself from autodigestion by the acid and pepsin that it produces?

There is copious production of mucus that forms a gel on the surface of the epithelium. Mixed within this is bicarbonate. Together, they ensure that the pH of the environment immediately adjacent to the epithelium is kept at neutral.

9. Describe the phases of gastric acid secretion.

- *Cephalic phase:* initiated by the thought, smell and taste of food. Leads to vagal activation that stimulates HCl and gastrin secretion
- *Gastric phase:* initiated by the presence of food in the stomach particularly protein rich food. There is, again, both an increase in the level of HCl *and* gastrin

▼

S

- *Intestinal phase:* initially, the presence of amino acid and food in the duodenum stimulate acid production. Later there is inhibition following the release of secretin and CCK

10. Summarise, then, the actions of gastrin.

- Stimulates gastric acid secretion
- Stimulates exocrine pancreatic secretions
- Stimulates gastric motility

STOMACH I

STOMACH II – APPLIED PHYSIOLOGY

1. Describe briefly the sources of gastric innervation.

- *Extrinsic supply:* from the sympathetic and parasympathetic systems
- *Intrinsic supply:* from the enteric nervous system

2. What is the autonomic supply?

- *Sympathetic:* from the cœliac plexus. Reduces gastric motility
- *Parasympathetic:* from the vagus nerve – causing increased motility

3. What is the storage capacity of the stomach?

1–2 L.

4. How does the stomach accommodate this volume without painful distension?

It undergoes the process of *receptive relaxation*. This is a vagally mediated reflex where the fundus and the body relax when distending with food.

5. Apart from receptive relaxation, name some other important gastric reflexes.

- *Peristalsis:* the *basic electrical rhythm* of the stomach generates *slow waves* that pass from inflow to outflow segments, propelling food
- *Retropulsion:* when chyme is pushed backwards and forwards in the lumen. This helps to break up boluses
- *Emptying*
- *Vomiting reflex*

6. List the hormones which stimulate gastric emptying.

- *Gastrin:* released from the gastric G-cells

- *CCK:* from the duodenum
- *Secretin:* also from the duodenum

7. What happens to the stomach during the process of vomiting? Outline the steps.

- The process begins with a deep inspiration
- This is followed by closure of the glottis
- There is diffuse contraction of the abdominal and thoracic muscles. This elevates the pressures of both compartments. The intra-abdominal pressure may rise to 800 mmHg
- Simultaneously, there is relaxation of the lower oesophageal sphincter
- There is a large retrograde contraction of the stomach, forcing the contents into the oesophagus following relaxation of the cricopharyngeus muscle
- There is generalised activity of the vasomotor centres, producing pallor and sweating. Also it is accompanied by tachycardia and palpitations
- Note that this process is coordinated by the *vomiting centre* of the medulla, and the chemoreceptor trigger zone (CRTZ)

8. Where is the CRTZ located, and what is its anatomic significance?

This is found in the area postrema in the floor of the 4th ventricle. Its position is significant because it lies outside of the BBB, and so can be influenced directly by noxious stimuli and drugs (such as opiates).

9. Briefly outline the physiological effects of pyloric stenosis.

- Persistent vomiting leads to dehydration which may lead to acute renal failure
- There is progressive metabolic alkalosis, which is perpetuated by the normal compensatory mechanisms

10. Describe how metabolic alkalosis develops in pyloric stenosis.

- Gastric secretions are rich in H^+ and Cl^-, both of which are lost
- There is a reduction of pancreatic exocrine secretions due to the reduced acid load at the duodenum. This therefore leads to retention of bicarbonate-rich pancreatic secretion, worsening the alkalosis already caused by loss of protons
- Volume depletion maintains the alkalosis by leading to bicarbonate absorption over chloride
- In order to maintain electrochemical neutrality, in response to loss of chloride, there is increased renal uptake of bicarbonate, further worsening the alkalosis

11. Describe some of the physiological effects of a total gastrectomy.

In simple terms, this leads to a complete loss of parietal cells leading to no gastric acid, together with no intrinsic factor nor pepsin:

- *No IF:* leads to vitamin B_{12} deficiency, manifest as a megaloblastic anaemia
- *Achlorhydria:* promotes iron deficiency
- *Dumping syndrome:* gastrectomy leads to the rapid transfer of hypertonic chyme into the small bowel. This leads to transfer of fluid from the extracellular space into the bowel. The immediate effect of this is abdominal distension, vomiting and diarrhoea. The fall in the circulating volume leads to the physiological shock response, with tachycardia, sweating and narrow pulse pressure
- *Hypokalaemia:* Vomitus contains around $10\,mmolL^{-1}$ of potassium, which is lost. Further potassium is lost from the kidney as protons are exchanged for potassium. Also, the increased aldosterone secreted by the adrenal cortex in response to fluid loss exacerbates renal potassium loss

SWALLOWING

1. Where is saliva produced?

- *Parotid glands:* produce a watery (serous) salivary secretion
- *Submandibular and sublingual glands:* the saliva produced contains a higher concentration of protein, and so is more mucinous
- *Oral glands:* smaller and spread diffusely

2. Give some normal values for their composition

The ionic composition of the saliva varies with the rate of secretion

- Na^+: 100 mmolL^{-1}
- Cl^-: 50 mmolL^{-1}
- K^+: 20 mmolL^{-1}
- HCO_3^-: 60 mmolL^{-1}
- Thus, there is less sodium and chloride in saliva than plasma, but more potassium and bicarbonate
- The saliva is *hypotonic* to plasma at all times. Its tonicity increases at higher flow rates, but it does not go beyond 70% of plasma tonicity

3. What is the principal digestive enzyme in saliva?

Salivary amylase (ptyalin), which breaks down starch into oligosaccharide molecules.

4. What is the volume of saliva produced daily?

This varies from 0.5–1.0 L per day.

5. How is the secretion controlled?

This is under the control of the ANS.

- *Parasympathetic stimulation:* produces a large volume of watery saliva that is low in protein
- *Sympathetic stimulation:* causes a reduction of secretion, with high mucin content

6. Describe the functions of saliva.

- Cleansing and protecting the mouth from harmful gastric acid and bile. Also has antibacterial properties due to the content of lysozyme
- Moistens food to allow for easy swallowing
- Enhancing the taste of food by dissolving food components and permitting more easy recognition by the taste buds
- Food digestion of carbohydrates, as mentioned above. Also involved in the digestion of fats – glandular secretions of the tongue contain lipase

7. What are the three basic phases of swallowing?

- Oral (or voluntary) phase
- Pharyngeal phase
- Oesophageal phase

8. What happens during the oral phase?

This is initiated voluntarily. The bolus of food is progressively moved upwards and backwards by pressure of the tongue against the hard palate. Once at the pharynx, the next phase is initiated. Note that this is the only voluntary phase of the swallowing reflex.

9. Describe what happens to the bolus in the pharyngeal phase.

- Contraction of the superior constrictor muscle of the pharynx elevates the soft palate and prevents food entering the nasopharynx
- The palatopharyngeal folds close in on one another, narrowing the aperture and preventing other boluses of food entering the pharynx
- The vocal folds come together. The larynx is pulled upwards and forwards against the epiglottis. This not only protects the airway, but stretches the top of the oesophagus and makes it more accommodating
- The upper oesophageal sphincter relaxes

▼

- The superior constrictor contracts, and food enters the oesophagus. This initiates a perilstaltic wave
- The medullary respiratory centre is inhibited

10. How is the food propagated down the oesophagus?

This final phase is called the *oesophageal phase.* The swallowing centre initiates a *primary* perilstaltic wave. This occurs together with relaxation of the lower oesophageal sphincter.

11. Then, what is a *secondary* perilstaltic wave?

If the primary coordinated perilstaltic wave fails to adequately clear the bolus of food, a vaso-vagal reflex is initiated that initiates a secondary wave of perilstalsis. This begins at the site of distension produced by the bolus, and moves down.

12. What is the normal resting pressure of the lower oesophageal sphincter?

30 mmHg. Note that lower sphincter is not a physical structure, but rather an area of high pressure in the lower oesophagus. Failure of normal relaxation during the oesophageal phase of swallowing underlies the pathophysiology of achalasia.

SYNAPSES I – THE NEUROMUSCULAR JUNCTION (NMJ)

1. Outline the stages of synaptic transmission.

- The action potential arrives at the presynaptic neurone, which causes the opening of voltage-gated Ca^{2+}-channels concentrated at the presynaptic membrane
- There is an influx of Ca^{2+} into the presynaptic terminal, increasing the intracellular $[Ca^{2+}]$. This is the trigger for the release of transmitter into the synaptic cleft by exocytosis
- Note that the neurotransmitter substance is stored in vesicles found at the nerve terminal. Each vesicle contains a 'quantum' of transmitter molecules
- The neurotransmitter diffuses across the synaptic cleft, and binds onto specific receptor proteins located on the postsynaptic membrane
- An action potential is generated in the postsynaptic cell
- The transmitter substance is degraded, and its component parts may be recycled through uptake at the presynatic nerve terminal

2. What are the names for the changes in membrane potential caused by binding of the transmitter to the synaptic receptors?

These transient changes in the membrane potential are called 'synaptic potentials'. A transient depolarisation of the postsynaptic cell is an 'excitatory postsynaptic potential' (EPSP). Similarly a transient hyperpolarisation is termed 'inhibitory postsynaptic potential' (IPSP).

3. What is meant by the terms 'temporal' and 'spatial' summation when referring to excitation of the postsynaptic membrane?

If the EPSP triggered by receptor binding is of sufficient magnitude, an action potential is triggered, with

▼

an influx of Na^+ or Ca^{2+}. This build up of EPSPs at the postsynaptic membrane is called 'summation'. It may occur through two mechanisms:

- *Temporal summation:* a rapid train of impulses from a single presynaptic cell causes EPSPs to add up, triggering an action potential in the postsynaptic cell
- *Spatial summation:* multiple presynatic neurones stimulate the postsynaptic cell simultaneously, leading to an accumulation of EPSPs, thus triggering an action potential

4. What is 'synaptic facilitation'?

This is where repeated stimulation of the presynaptic neurone causes a progressive rise in the amplitude of the postsynaptic response. It arises from a local accumulation of Ca^{2+} at the presynaptic terminal and is an example of short-term synaptic plasticity.

5. How many NMJs may a skeletal muscle fibre have?

Despite its long length, each skeletal muscle fibre has only one neurone committed to it. Thus, there is only one NMJ per fibre.

6. What is the neurotransmitter at the NMJ, and what is the source of this chemical?

Acetylcholine (ACh). Intra-cellular choline combines with the acetyl group of acetyl-Coenzyme A. The catalyst for this reaction is the cytosolic enzyme choline acetyltransferase (CAT).

7. How is this chemical removed from the NMJ following release into the synaptic cleft?

Following unbinding from postsynaptic cholinoceptors, ACh undergoes hydrolysis into acetate and choline. This degradation is catalysed by the enzyme acetylcholinesterase (AChE). Choline is then recycled back into the presynaptic terminal for further ACh production.

8. Generally speaking, how may the cholinergic receptors be classified?

Cholinergic receptors may be *Nicotinic* or *Muscarinic.*

9. What is their distribution in the body?

- *Nicotinic:* found at the NMJ, ANS ganglia, and at various points in the central nervous system (CNS). They are connected directly to ion channels for rapid cellular activation
- *Muscarinic:* found at postganglionic parasympathetic synapses (e.g. heart, smooth muscles and glandular tissue), in the CNS and gastric parietal cells. They are G-protein coupled, leading to either activation of phospholipase C, direct activation of K^+-channels, or inhibition of adenylate cyclase

SYNAPSES II – MUSCARINIC PHARMACOLOGY

1. Name some drugs that activate muscarinic cholinoceptors. What are these compounds used for?

These may be of two broad types based on the mechanism of muscarinic activation:

- *Through direct stimulation:* examples include *carbachol*, *bethanechol* and *pilocarpine. Bethanechol* has been used for the management of postoperative paralytic ileus and urinary retention. *Pilocarpine* is used for the management of closed angle glaucoma

- *Through indirect stimulation: anticholiesterases* promote increased cholinergic stimulation by preventing the hydrolysis of ACh at the synapse. Examples include *neostigmine* and *edrophonium* (both quaternary ammonium compounds). Note that these agents are used therapeutically for the reversal of neuromuscular (nicotinic cholinoceptors) blockade. However, as a side effect of preventing ACh hydrolysis, they may also increase the activity of muscarinic cholinoceptors, e.g. at autonomic ganglia

2. What physiologic effects does stimulation of muscarinic receptors lead to?

Essentially, there is increased activation of the PNS:

- *Cardiac:* with negative inotropic and chronotropic effects, with a reduction in the arterial pressure. This latter effect is exacerbated through peripheral vasodilatation

- *Increased glandular secretion:* such as increased bronchial, salivary and mucosal secretion. Also increased lacrimation

- *Increased smooth muscle contraction:* such as in the gut and bronchi. Increased bronchial secretions exacerbate the pathologic effects of bronchoconstriction

- *Eye changes:* see below

3. Outline the effects of muscarinic stimulation in the eye.

Stimulation leads two main parasympathetic effects:

- Contraction of the *constrictor pupillae* muscle, reducing the size of the pupil. This also has the effect of improving the drainage of the aqueous humour in those with raised intraocular pressure. In this respect, *pilocarpine*, a muscarinic agonist, has been used for closed angle glaucoma
- Contraction of the ciliary muscles, leading to accommodation for near vision by changing the shape of the lens

4. What class of drug is atropine?

Atropine is a muscarinic cholinoceptor antagonist. It is a tertiary amine, so undergoes gut absorption, and CNS penetration.

5. What are its physiologic effects?

Its effects may be understood in terms of parasympathetic inhibition:

- *Cardiovascular:* although it produces tachycardia due to parasympathetic inhibition, a low dose may initially give rise to a *bradycardia* due to central vagal activation. Ultimately, the resulting tachycardia is only mild, since the cardiac parasympathetic tone is inhibited without any concurrent sympathetic stimulation
- *Gut:* decreased gut motility, leading to constipation
- *Relaxation of other smooth muscles:* such as in the bronchi. May also lead to urinary retention due to its effects on the bladder
- *Inhibition of glandular secretions:* such as salivary and bronchial secretions
- *Pupiliary dilatation (mydriasis) and failure of accommodation:* leads to blurred vision and photophobia
- *CNS:* causes excitation, restlessness and agitation

6. Why have agents in the same class as atropine been used for premedication prior to induction of anaesthesia?

- Reduction of bronchial and salivary secretions prior to intubation reduces the risk of aspiration
- Prevention of bronchospasm during intubation through relaxation of the bronchial smooth muscle
- *Inducing drowsiness preoperatively: hyoscine* (unlike atropine) causes drowsiness and some amnesia
- *Antiemesis:* especially *hyoscine*
- Reduction of the unwanted effects of *neostigmine* (used for reversal of paralysis) – such as increased salivation and bradycardia
- Counteraction of the hypotensive and bradycardic effects of some inhaled anaesthetic agents

7. Therefore, in summary, list the uses of these agents.

Uses include:

- Premedication prior to anaesthesia, e.g. *glycopyrronium, hyoscine*
- Reversal of bradycardia, e.g. *atropine* for vaso-vagal attacks or during cardio-pulmonary resuscitation
- Anti-spasmodic for the gut, e.g. *hyoscine*
- Anti-emesis, e.g. *hyoscine* for motion sickness
- Mydriatic for eye examination, e.g. *atropine, tropicamide*
- *Organophosphate* poisoning, e.g. atropine. These agents are potent anticholinesterases

SYNAPSES III – NICOTINIC PHARMACOLOGY

1. From a pharmacological point of view, where are the two most important locations of nicotinic cholinoceptors?

Although found throughout the CNS, the two most clinically important areas for nicotinic cholinoceptors are at autonomic ganglia (serving both the SNS and PNS), and at the postsynaptic membrane of the NMJ.

2. Name some agents that block nicotinic cholinoceptors at the NMJ. What uses do they have?

Agents include:

- *Non-depolarising block*
  - Tubocurarine
  - Vecuronium
  - Pancuronium
  - Gallamine
- *Depolarising block*
  - Suxamethonium
- It follows that these agents are used for producing muscular paralysis during induction and maintenance of anaesthesia. Note that the non-depolarising drugs are *quaternary ammonium* compounds, so are not absorbed by the gut

3. What is meant by a 'depolarising' and a 'non-depolarising' block?

- Non-depolarising block is where there is competitive antagonism of ACh at the motor endplates. Thus, these agents act as a physical barrier to muscle fibre activation
- Depolarising block is where there is an initial rapid and sustained activation of the postsynaptic membrane until finally there is loss of excitability and the block established

- Therefore with a depolarising block, there is an initial muscular fasciculation until the block is established
- Despite this, the depolarising agents produce a more rapid onset of block than the non-depolarising agents

4. Outline some of the unwanted effects associated with depolarising agents.

- *Muscular pain:* following the use of *suxamethonium*, patients often report generalised or localised muscle pain. This is related to the initial painful fasciculation produced by this agent as part of its depolarising block
- *Hyperkalaemia:* due to loss of potassium from the muscle fibre. This occurs because of the increases in sodium uptake that occur during the depolarising block causes a net loss of potassium from the cell
- *Malignant hyperthermia:* an autosomal dominant condition, leading to a rapid and uncontrolled hyperthermia following a depolarising block and fasciculation
- Bradycardia in the case of suxamethonium due to a direct muscarinic stimulation

5. How may the block at the NMJ be reversed?
Non-depolarising agents may be reversed by the use of anticholinesterases.

As the name suggests, the AChEs prevent the hydrolysis of ACh at the synaptic cleft. The local increase in the concentration of ACh is enough to overcome the competitive block produced by the non-depolarising agents.

6. Name some of these agents. What uses do they have?
Examples of anticholinesterases include: *neostigmine, physostigmine and edrophonium.*

Apart from use in the reversal of non-depolarising muscle relaxants, they have also been used for the diagnosis and palliation of myasthenia gravis. In this condition, there is an immune-mediated destruction of ACh receptors, leading to progressive muscular weakness.

7. What is the danger of using anticholinesterase agents with depolarising neuromuscular blockers?

By causing a local increase of ACh, the anticholinesterase agents exacerbate the block produced by depolarising muscle relaxants.

8. What happens to the characteristics of the block caused by depolarising agents with continuous administration?

The initial depolarising block produced is also termed a 'phase I block'. With repeated administration, a 'phase II' block is encountered, when a non-depolarising block occurs. This phenomenon of depolarising agents is also known as a DUAL BLOCK, and can lead to prolonged paralysis.

Therefore, given the change in the characteristics of the block, during phase II, the action of depolarising agents may be terminated with the use of anticholinesterases.

THYROID GLAND

1. What is the basic histologic structure of the thyroid gland?

- The thyroid is composed of numerous follicles that have a central fluid-filled cavity. They are lined with follicular cells that secrete the main hormones
- Interspersed among the follicles are the para-follicular cells

2. Which hormones does the thyroid produce?

- *Tetra-iodothyronine (T_4, thyroxine):* the principle hormone of the thyroid gland
- *Tri-iodothyronine (T_3):* measure for measure, this is more potent than T_4, however, has a shorter duration of action
- *Calcitonin:* produced by the para-follicular cells. This is important in the regulation of serum calcium *(see 'Calcium balance')*

3. Name another source of T_3 other than the thyroid.

This may also be produced by the conversion of T_4 in the peripheral tissues. In fact, the thyroid accounts for only 20% of the extrathyroid pool of T_3.

4. Which other hormone may be produced following the peripheral conversion of T_4?

Reversed-T_3 (r-T_3). This is an inactive hormone acts as a point of peripheral thyroid hormone control.

5. Outline the steps involved in the production of T_3 and T_4.

- *Iodide trapping:* dietary iodine is concentrated into the follicular cells by an active pump mechanism
- *Oxidation:* of iodide to a reactive form by the enzyme peroxidase. This is located on the apical membrane

- *Organification:* through binding with amino acids – mainly tyrosine. These form tyrosyl units
- *Thyroglobulin formation:* tyrosyl units combine with a protein core to form thyroglobulin
- *Internal coupling:* tyrosyl units combine on the thyroglobulin molecule to form T_3 or T_4 molecules still bound to the protein core
- *Storage:* the thyroglobulin molecules are transferred to the colloid of the follicles for storage
- *Release:* this occurs following stimulation by thyroid-stimulating hormone (TSH). The thyroglobulin molecule is taken up into the follicle by endocytosis, and following fusion with lysosomes, releases the T_3 and T_4 molecules

6. How are the molecules transported in the circulation?

- T_4: predominantly bound to thyroid-binding globulin, and a smaller proportion to thyroid-binding prealbumin. A small fraction is unbound
- T_3: bound mainly to thyroid-binding globulin. A higher proportion is found unbound

7. Outline the basic physiological roles of thyroid hormone.

- *Increased BMR:* this leads to increased oxygen consumption and increased heat production
- *Protein metabolism:* this has implications for growth and development. Both protein formation and degradation are enhanced. During hormone excesses, degradation is increased over synthesis
- *Carbohydrate metabolism:* all aspects of metabolism are increased-cellular uptake of glucose, glycolysis, gluconeogenesis and glycogenolysis
- *Fat metabolism:* lead to lipolysis with a concomitant increase in the plasma FFA concentration. At the same time increases the cellular oxidation of these fatty acids

- *Others systems:* increases the CO, in part through increasing the BMR and by enhancing the effects of other hormones. Also important for CNS development and increasing cortical arousal
- *Potentiation of other hormones:* enhances the actions of catacholamines and insulin, among others

8. What is their mechanism of action?
Like steroid hormones, the thyroid hormones act through an intracellular mechanism. They penetrate the cytoplasm with ease and act on intracellular receptors to active various genes in the cell's nucleus.

9. How is hormone production regulated?
The anterior pituitary hormone TSH controls release of hormone. It enhances all of the steps of thyroid hormone production outlined above. Various other hormones stimulate release, such as estrogens.

10. Other than a goitre, what other physical signs may you expect to find when examining a patient with Grave's disease?
- Generally, may have features of recent weight loss
- Patient may be flushed, suggesting heat intolerance
- *Other features of sympathetic stimulation:* peripheral tremor, presence of atrial fibrillation
- *Extrathyroid manifestations:* eye signs, thyroid acropachy (a form of pseudo-clubbing of the fingers) and pretibial myxoedema

11. What are the eye signs?
- *Lid retraction and lid lag:* due to increased sympathetic activation of the levator palpebrae superiorus
- *Exophthalmos/proptosis:* due to oedema of the retro-orbital fat
- *Diplopia:* due to combinations of the above

THYROID GLAND

VALSALVA MANOEUVRE

1. What is the Valsalva manoeuvre?

This is forced expiration against a closed glottis.

2. In which situations may it occur during everyday life?

Examples include:

- Coughing
- Straining to lift a heavy weight
- Straining at defecation

3. Below is a diagram of the changes in the arterial pressure and heart rate during the Valsalva manoeuvre. Explain the step-by-step changes that occur in these physiological parameters.

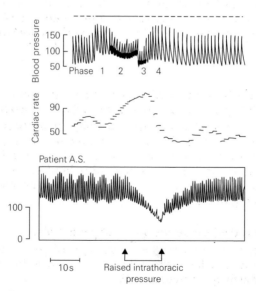

From Levick JR. An Introduction to Cardiovascular Physiology, 1990, Butterworth Heinemann

- *Phase I:* The changes are initiated by a rise in the intrathoracic pressure (i.e. becomes less negative)
- This causes pressure upon the thoracic aorta, which produces a transient rise in the arterial pressure
- *Phase II:* Following this, there is a progressive fall in the MAP and pulse pressure. This occurs because the rise in the intrathoracic pressure reduces the venous return to the right atrium, leading to a fall in the stroke volume and hence the CO through the Frank-Starling mechanism
- The fall in the MAP induces a reflex tachycardia. This, together with peripheral vasoconstriction put a halt on a further fall in the arterial pressure
- *Phase III:* Following opening of the glottis during cessation of the manoeuvre, there is a sudden drop in the arterial pressure as the direct pressure on the thoracic aorta is relieved
- *Phase IV:* This fall in the intrathoracic pressure soon improves the venous return. This produces a rise in the arterial pressure. This pressure rise stimulates baroreceptors, which gives rise to a reflex bradycardia

4. What is the practical use of testing a person's physiological response during the Valsalva manoeuvre?

This is a test of autonomic function, e.g. in those with diabetes mellitus. In cases of autonomic neuropathy, there is a sustained fall in the arterial pressure for as long as the manoeuvre is held. Also, in phase IV, there is no overshoot rise of the arterial pressure and no resulting braycardia.

5. Has this manoeuvre any therapeutic role?

It has been used in the termination of paroxysms of supraventricular tachycardia since there is increased vagal activity during phase IV.

V

VALSALVA MANOEUVRE

V VENOUS PRESSURE

1. Draw the waveform of the CVP, labelling the various deflections.

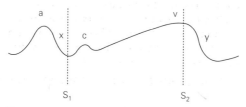

The jugular venous pulse waveform in relation to the first (S_1) and second (S_2) heart sounds.

2. What do the individual deflections represent?

- *a* wave is due to atrial contraction
- *x* wave follows the end of atrial systole
- *c* wave is produced by bulging of the tricuspid valve into the atrium at the start of ventricular systole
- *v* wave occurs due to progressive venous return to the atrium. It indicates the timing of ventricular systole, but is not directly caused by it
- *y* descent occurs following opening of the tricuspid valve

3. Why are the veins considered to be the main 'capacitance vessels' of the body?

The body's veins and venules are thin-walled and voluminous, and so are capable of accommodating much of the circulating blood volume. In fact, about 2/3 of the blood volume is to be found in the venous system.

4. What is the normal range for the CVP?

0–10 mmHg.

V

5. Which factors determine the venous return to the heart, and hence the CVP?

- *Circulating blood volume:* it follows that the greater the blood volume, the greater the venous pressure

- *Venous tone:* sympathetic stimulation in various peripheral and visceral venous beds causes venoconstriction, leading to increased venous return and venous pressure. This is an important compensatory mechanism in hypovolaemia that maintains the stroke volume and CO

- *Posture:* supine posture or leg elevation increases the venous return

- *Skeletal muscle pump:* the calf pump system is particularly important in increasing the venous return during exercise, when muscle contraction compresses the deep soleus plexus of veins

- *Respiratory cycle and intrathoracic pressure:* during inspiration, the intrathoracic pressure falls (i.e. becomes more negative) increasing the venous return gradient to the heart. The opposite occurs during expiration

V

VENTILATION/PERFUSION RELATIONSHIPS

1. On which factors does adequate blood oxygenation depend on?

- *Normal ventilation of the lung:* this is determined by a normal respiratory drive and a functionally normal respiratory apparatus (includes the brain, chest wall, airways and lung parenchyma)
- Adequate diffusion of respiratory gasses across the alveolar wall
- Matching of ventilation and perfusion

2. By what process do the respiratory gases pass through the various anatomic barriers to pass into the blood?

Through diffusion.

3. Which physical law determines diffusion across membranes?

Fick's law of diffusion: This states that the amount of gas diffusing per unit time (i.e. the rate of diffusion) is *inversely* proportional to the thickness of the barrier and *directly* proportional to the surface area of the barrier.

4. What are the anatomic layers that respiratory gases have to pass through to reach the haemoglobin molecule in the red cells?

- *The fluid lining the alveoli:* gases initially dissolve in this before proceeding to the next layer
- *Alveolar epithelium* and through its basement membrane
- *Interstitial space:* which also contains fluid
- Basement membrane of capillary endothelium
- Capillary endothelium

▼

- Plasma
- Red cell membrane

5. What is shunt?
This refers to venous blood that passes to the systemic circulation without first being oxygenated in the lungs.

6. Is this always pathological?
No, under normal circumstances, 1–2% of the CO bypasses the alveoli. This is called the anatomic shunt.

7. Where are the sites for normal anatomic shunt?
- The bronchial circulation
- *Cardiac Thebesian veins:* that drain coronary venous blood directly into the left side of the heart

8. Is there also some normal shunt though the lungs?
Yes, this occurs in some lung units that have a low V/Q ratio – i.e. poorly ventilated units that are well perfused. This increases in various disease states.

9. What is meant by the term *venous admixture*?
This is the total shunt derived from normal anatomic shunt and the shunt arising from lung units with a low V/Q ratio.

10. How else may pathological shunting arise?
From right to left shunting through the heart, typically occurring with cyanotic septal defects such as tetralogy of Fallot.

11. What is the effect of venous admixture on the arterial saturations of oxygen and carbon dioxide?
There is a reduction of the PaO_2 with little effect on the $PaCO_2$ due to differences in the shapes of their respective

dissociation curves. The effect on the PaO_2 can be seen as an increase in the alveolar-arterial PO_2 difference.

12. What is the overall V/Q ratio of the normal lung?

In the steady state, the ventilation-perfusion ratio is normally 0.8 for the entire lung. At the two extreme ends of the V/Q spectrums are:

- *Wasted ventilation:* in the lung units that are ventilated but not perfused. The V/Q is infinite
- *Pure shunt:* in the lung units which are perfused but not ventilated, where the V/Q is zero

It can be seen that at both ends of the spectrum, there is a fall in the PaO_2. The ideal lung unit has ventilation and perfusion well matched – i.e. where the V/Q is close to 1.

13. How do ventilation and perfusion vary in different parts of the lung?

- The lower parts of the lung are better perfused than the higher parts
- The lower parts are also relatively better ventilated. (The lower portions of the lung lie on a steeper portion of the compliance curve than the apex)
- However, in terms of the ratio of the two variables, the V/Q falls going from the apex to the base of the lung

14. You have stated that adequate oxygenation depends on an even matching of ventilation and perfusion in the various lung units. How is the ratio kept as even as possible?

There are two main mechanisms by which mismatching of ventilation and perfusion is kept to the minimum in lung units:

- *Hypoxic vasoconstriction:* a fall in the PaO_2 that accompanies a fall in the V/Q leads to reflex vasoconstriction of pulmonary arterioles. This evens out the V/Q, improving oxygenation. Conversely, if the V/Q is high, there is pulmonary vasodilatation, again matching the V/Q

- *Changes in bronchial smooth muscle tone:* this is also sensitive to hypoxaemia, altering the calibre of the airways and therefore ventilation of lung units

15. Give some causes for hypoxaemia due to a V/Q mismatch.

- Congenital cardiac defects mentioned above
- Pneumonia
- Pulmonary oedema, e.g due to cardiac failure and ARDS
- Pulmonary embolism
- Brochiectasis, asthma

Note that this produces a Type I respiratory failure. Hyperventilation does not increase the PaO_2 due to the large shunt, but it blows off the CO_2. Thus, there is hypoxaemia, with a low or normal $PaCO_2$.

16. Therefore, summarise the four general causes of hypoxia.

- *Alveolar hypoventilation:* leading to a *Type II* respiratory failure with elevated $PaCO_2$
- *Diffusion abnormalities:* seen as an abnormal transfer factor, e.g. in diffuse pulmonary fibrosis
- *Shunt:* blood passes from the right to left heart without being oxygenated by the lung, e.g. in cyanotic congenital heart disease
- *Ventilation-perfusion mismatch:* when the ratio of the two is greater or less than one, the blood returning to the heart in the pulmonary veins will be hypoxaemic. Hypoxia due to such a mismatch constitutes a *Type I* respiratory failure